The Male
Stress
Syndrome

Also by the Author

The Female Stress Syndrome: How to Become Stress-Wise in the '90s

Beyond Quick Fixes: Control Your Irresistible Urges Before They Control You

Passions: Manage Despair, Fear, Rage & Guilt and Heighten Your Capacity for Joy, Love, Hope & Awe

THE MALE
STRESS
SYNDROME

How to Survive Stress in the '90s

Second Edition

GEORGIA WITKIN, Ph.D.

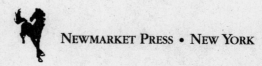

NEWMARKET PRESS • NEW YORK

None of the "patients" discussed in this book are based on any one individual. All names are fictitious and all case histories are the author's creation based on the composite of her professional experience.

Second Edition
94 95 96 97   10 9 8 7 6 5 4 3 2 1

Library of Congress Cataloging-in-Publication Data

Witkin, Georgia.
    The male stress syndrome: how to survive stress in the '90s / Georgia Witkin-Lanoil. — 2nd ed.
        p.   cm.
    Includes bibliographical references and index.
    ISBN 1-55704-206-3 (hc)
    ISBN 1-55704-205-5 (pb)
    1. Stress (Psychology). 2. Men—Psychology. 3. Stress management. I. Title.
BF575.S75W59   1994
155.980428081—dc20   94-27468
                                                            CIP

Quantity Purchases

Companies, professional groups, clubs, and other organizations may qualify for special terms when ordering quantities of this title. For information, contact Newmarket Press, Special Sales Department, 18 East 48th Street, New York, NY 10017, or call 212-832-3575.

Manufactured in the United States of America.

Contents

Acknowledgments

I WOULD LIKE THIS TO BE A DEDICATION TO THE FOLLOWING SPECIAL PEOPLE who have reduced *my* stress through their support for this project.

To Esther Margolis, Keith Hollaman, Grace Farrell, and Mia Oberlink for their commitment to this book.

To Robert Benjamin, Chief of the Communicable Disease Bureau, Alameda County, California, and my dear friend since the day I was born, who so generously reviewed each chapter for medical accuracy and contributed many new points of view.

To Dr. Stanley Fisher, College of Physicians and Surgeons, Columbia University, and my wise colleague, who helped to shape the direction of this research with his clinical insights.

To all my parents, my family, and to my daughter, Kimberly Hope, for their love.

And to all stressed men and the women who love them.

The Male
Stress
Syndrome

INTRODUCTION

I WAS RECENTLY ASKED ON *20/20* WHY SO MANY MEN AVOID DOCTORS. After all, for more than three decades we have been bombarded with information about the life-threatening effects of stress on men. Men have been frightened by their risk of heart attack, ulcers, and high blood pressure. They worry each day about their diet, their exercises, or their lack of exercise. They try hard to give up smoking and to reduce their drinking. They calculate their life expectancy, and then recalculate it, pretending that they *have* given up smoking and reduced their drinking. They worry about stress, and then worry about worrying.

So it's not that men don't know that stress can affect their bodies and their behavior, but that they're not fully convinced that it's doing its damage *now*. They admit that stress will have an effect someday, but not today. They haven't had a heart attack or a stroke today; they don't have an ulcer today, or high blood pressure—so today they are okay. Tomorrow, they say, they will do something about stress. But the effects of stress today are what cause the problems of tomorrow.

Men often haven't been told why they develop certain stress symptoms, why they are particularly vulnerable or sensitive to certain types of stresses, or how they can help themselves, their fathers, and their sons. They are told about stress perils, but need to learn about stress origins and stress management.

The Male Stress Syndrome is a book for these men and for

the women who love them. It is certainly not the first book you have encountered on stress, but it is different from others in many ways. First, it grew directly out of the response from men and women who have read my book *The Female Stress Syndrome*, which identifies the stresses and stress symptoms that are uniquely or more frequently female. Although many stresses and symptoms are shared by men and women, I describe in *The Female Stress Syndrome* those that women have as their own. For example, women are more likely to develop depression, migraine headaches, eating disorders, and anxiety attacks than are men. They have reproductive system problems, such as premenstrual tension, irregularities of the menstrual cycle, and paramenopausal dysfunctions, which are aggravated by stress, that men, of course, will never have. Women must cope with the life changes involved with becoming a wife, or mother, or both, during a time of high divorce rates and low economic stability. They deal with aging in a youth-beauty culture and face the widowhood epidemic. They can claim the stresses of tokenism, glass ceilings, and sexism, and, often, years of nonassertiveness training. Together, these stresses and stress symptoms make up what I call the Female Stress Syndrome, and I show readers of *The Female Stress Syndrome* how to identify and manage these stresses, live with them, or make them go away. Surely, these readers have questioned, there must be stresses and symptoms that are uniquely or more frequently suffered by men as well.

Yes, there are. Although heart attacks at younger ages and high blood pressure are obvious male stress symptoms, many symptoms are less obvious. Physical symptoms, such as muscle aches and tension headaches, are often ignored or easily passed off as the flu or fatigue. Psychological symptoms, such as disorganization and decision-making difficulties, generally are neither recognized nor explained. These and other male stresses and symptoms are treated as "facts of life" by too many men, and silently do their dangerous damage.

The Male Stress Syndrome also differs from other books on

stress in that information has been gathered not only from men, but from women as well. The research literature that exists to date contains study after study focusing on men's reports about their daily stresses and symptoms. But the investigators usually have not been direct observers of their subjects' stress, and the subjects themselves are often unwilling to recognize all the stresses and stress symptoms in their lives, as we'll discover in this book. The women around them, however, are often most observant, providing many insights into male stress that have not emerged in the studies done up to this point.

For the original edition of this book, I created a Male Stress Survey that I administered over a six-month period to more than five hundred men, selected at random and representing some forty different occupations, from mechanic, graduate student, actor, and police officer, to advertising executive, teacher, psychiatrist, and small-business owner. I also gave a similar survey to hundreds of the women they were close to—mothers, wives, sisters, daughters, and friends. Respondents were asked to identify the men's stressors, stress behaviors, and physical signs of stress, and to expand on how they feel or act in a variety of stressful situations. The women often provided information that added to, rather than contradicted, the data gathered from their men. And their observations were surprisingly consistent, regardless of the kinds of work the men did or the different life-styles they led.

Of course, the original research and survey results alone are not enough to tell us about today's male stress, so in this second edition I include current case studies about real men living real lives. The patterns stay the same! We hear them talk about the pressures of open competition, which starts as early as Little League and is no less stressful in the occupational big leagues. Men speak of performance anxieties from the time they get out of bed in the morning to go to work to the time they get back into bed to relax and play. They talk about their need for a sense of control over their own lives, with their jobs, with their children, and even with their wives. They talk about the need for achievement, which drives them ahead, and the fear of failure and layoffs, which holds them back—and the conflict when they are caught between the two.

Some of the case study material in this book comes from the decade of stress management workshops that I have conducted with police, firefighters, teachers, unions, nurses and hospital workers, students, patients, executives, and management and labor groups. Some of it comes from in-depth interviews I conducted for this book with fifty men of all ages in different stages of life change, who generously (and anonymously) shared their most private experiences. Some of the case study material represents a composite of information that my clinical patients have shared with me over the years.

"What's a Type A?" they asked me. "Because I think I am one!"

"What's the matter with me?" they asked. "I hate to wait and I'm always running late."

"What's another birthday?" they asked. "Why do I care so much?"

Male stresses, whether obvious, subtle, or hidden, seem to fall into one of four focus areas:

- *Body concerns.* Height, weight, and athletic prowess count when you are a boy (particularly height, say all studies). Add to those elements a concern about sexual functioning when you are a young man, and about stamina when you are middle-aged. Health is your major concern after that. And for good reason. Although men are strong, they do not necessarily live long. More men than women are conceived, but the male fetal mortality rate is higher than that for females—and the mortality pattern does not change throughout the lifespan. By the time men are over sixty-five, women outnumber them by 33 percent!

- *Career concerns.* From his earliest awareness, many a

man wrestles with the question of what he wants to be when he grows up. Not *who* he wants to be or *how* he wants to be, but *what* he wants to be. His occupations and the preparation for it can become his preoccupation. His source of income often becomes his source of public identity, and his economic success becomes his measure of self-worth. He is taught to provide and produce, to make choices, and to be in control. When his work circumstances are unpredictable or beyond his control, when achievement feedback is not forthcoming, when his expectations are not realistic—stress! And when it's appropriate to give up control and he cannot—more stress!

• *Family concerns.* What is it like to become a husband after two decades or more of training as a son? What is it like to become a father once, twice, or three times within the same decade in which you have become a wage earner, taxpayer, and homeowner? What is it like to have to "visit" with your own children while you are living with someone else's? Being a family man in the 1990s can be far from predictable, and can make many extra demands, both physically and psychologically.

• *Personal concerns.* Competitive compulsions, age/career deadlines, pressures to provide, and fears of impotence, illness, and death are common male stresses. Unfortunately, most men do not know how common they are! Years of being told to "be a man" and "stand on your own two feet" can lead to years of stoicism and emotional channeling or withdrawal. Setting a good example is seen to be more important than settling a bad conflict within yourself. Having confidence is seen to be more important than having confidants. Going it alone, apparently, precludes going for therapy. In fact, many men I interviewed listed therapy, along with surgery and death, as their major fears. Without communication, personal concerns soon develop into private problems, which in turn preoccupy and further isolate men under stress.

Perhaps the most urgent question my *Female Stress Syndrome* readers asked me was, "What can I do if I am living with a stressed man?" Perhaps the most urgent question I can ask you is, "What can you do if that stressed man is *you*?" The answer to both questions starts with stress knowledge. In this book, you'll gain knowledge about the sources and consequences of male stress—and knowledge is power. With knowledge you can make use of early warning signals and recognize fully the pressures of work, family, and society, and their effect on you physically and psychologically. Equally important, you'll learn both short- and long-term techniques to relieve and help manage your stresses, to make living with the Male Stress Syndrome a bit easier.

1 BATTLE OF THE STRESSES: UNDERSTANDING MALE/FEMALE DIFFERENCES

MEN AND WOMEN SHARE SO MUCH. THEY LAUGH TOGETHER, LOVE together, work together, play together, stay together. Both sexes experience infatuation, rage, and despair. They both suffer daily indignities and lifelong inevitabilities: they share traffic jams, computer errors, parents aging, and children changing. But too often they have no knowledge of each other's particular stresses. Men may view many women's health complaints as "attention-getters" rather than tension tell-tales. Women, on the other hand, may secretly suspect that ailments frequently suffered by men are minor discomforts compared to premenstrual symptoms, pregnancy, childbirth, and menopause. Men say that chauffeuring, grocery shopping, and entertaining sound like easy busywork; women claim they will trade these chores anytime for "men's" activities, like washing the car.

Actually, men's and women's lives may be equally stressful, but many of the stressors and symptoms are indeed different. Women are in a kind of double jeopardy for stress symptoms, because they have a reproductive system that both creates stress and is vulnerable to the effects of stress. For example, they are susceptible to menstrual disorders, migraine headaches, anxiety attacks, depression, and eating disorders such as anorexia (a compulsion to exercise control by not eating) and bulimia (gorging and, often, purging food). Men, however, find themselves at a higher risk of *earlier fatality* from their stress symptoms. These, as we'll discuss in detail in later chapters, include high blood pressure, high cholesterol, heart attacks, alcoholism, and peptic ulcers. And adding insult to injury are sexual dysfunctions such as premature ejaculation and erectile problems.

The stresses and stress symptoms caused by different psychologies, behavior models, kinds of life change, peer and parent pressures, and cultural reinforcements are quite different for men and women as well. In this chapter we'll take a look at some of these, and set the stage for much of the stress information that follows. Most important, I hope that this chapter will remind us that the question is not "Who has it worse?" but, rather, "How can we help each other make it better?"

STRESS CLOCKS

For both men and women, the passage of time can itself be stressful. It reminds us that there are realities of life beyond our control, and low control leads to high stress. It brings uncertainties, and a low factor of predictability leads to high stress. It brings change, and low stability leads again to high stress. But for both men and women, the passage of time has another, more personal, meaning. For women, it is often that their *biological clock* is running "too fast."

For men, on the other hand, birthdays can make them feel that their *achievement clock* is running "too slow." This difference suggests more than different priorities—it reflects different realities. A study of nearly three million death certificates for people who had died of natural causes shows that men are more likely to die in the week *before* their birthdays than in any other week of the year. This astounding discovery suggests that men use birthdays as an occasion to take stock of their accomplishments. If they haven't reached their expectations, their very survival may be affected.

Men can have their first family in their teens, start another family a decade later, father even more children in their middle years, and continue to produce progeny into old age. Women, however, go through menopause in their late forties and early fifties, and that biological clock cannot be reset. If a woman delayed starting a family to pursue a career, she may find she's under pregnancy pressure by her middle thirties.

Some men, of course, experience fertility problems, and find them a source of stress: passing on a family name, family business, or family pride are important achievements to most men. If infertility is a problem for them, they can feel that their own body has betrayed them. More often, however, there is no fertility problem, and achievements other than those attached to a family preoccupy men. By certain ages they would like to achieve certain positions, salaries, or kinds of recognition. Decade birthdays seem to be particularly important measurements of success for men. If they approach those round numbers with no sign of the achievements they expected, their families may begin to notice signs of depression, disinterest in work, or even despair. If they are even more successful than they had expected, on the other hand, they may want—and enjoy—a gala fiftieth birthday party. Think about it. How many women, concerned as they are about aging, get a huge surprise fiftieth birthday party? How many would want one?

GOALS, GAMES, AND GUILT

The need for achievement seems to be as universal among all adults, male or female, as is the need for mastery among infants and children. The same drive that pushes toddlers to run, reach, and catch pushes adults to continually up their own quotas for themselves. However, the stresses that men and women encounter along the way to achievement, and even after achievement, are quite different.

One male/female difference concerns competition. From their earliest days, boys are taught the rules of the competition game. They play such games among themselves, choosing up sides and fighting battles for a tree, a hill, or a swing. They are encouraged to join organized baseball teams and boy scout troops. They are told to play fair, but to win, win, win. Their team is counting on them, their parents are watching them, and their friends are cheering for them. They learn games of chance—how to bluff and how to finesse. They learn dating games—how to "score" and what it means to "strike out." Listen to the language of business, says author Betty Lehan Harragan, and you'll hear the language of gamesmanship that has been learned young:*

"Let's take the ball and run with it."
"Go for it!"
"See if it 'plays.'"
"One for *our* team!"

In a recent study of executive women conducted by marketing professor Carol Scott, respondents complained that sports are still the main basis of affectional relations among men at work—an area from which the women are routinely excluded.

This early and constant exposure to competition has both a functional and dysfunctional effect. It is functional in that men are prepared to fight their way up the corporate ladder or through a tough day on the job. As a group they believe, according to the Male Stress Survey I conducted for this book,

*For further information on the references and specific studies cited throughout this book, see the Bibliography, beginning on page 209.

that hard work pays off and that being "one of the boys" is more desirable than being the boss's Number One. It is dysfunctional and stress-producing in that men often develop into *compulsive competitors*. Even when they no longer have to compete with others for a job or promotion, they compete with themselves. If this time they were excellent, then next time they have to be even better. Better than their father might have been, better than *they* ever thought they would be.

Women are more likely to be *closet competitors*. Many generations of women were taught that sugar and spice were nice and that the thrill of victory was less satisfying than silent sacrifice and service. Does this mean that the drive for mastery and the goal of success is less common among women than men? No. But it does mean that women are more likely to try to hide their competitive feelings and efforts than men. They observe the activities of other women and then up their quotas for themselves. If the head of the PTA is also a real estate broker *and* bakes her own cookies, then she may have unknowingly set a new standard for many of her female friends. Quiet competition like this is also never-ending, as there is always one more demand a woman can make on herself.

A surprising male/female difference that surfaced in the hundreds of interviews I conducted for both books involves the type of guilt fallout associated with achievement. For men, there is shame and guilt associated with lack of success and low job satisfaction. For women, guilt is often associated with public success and high job satisfaction. Here is why:

When they are asked to identify themselves, men most frequently refer to their occupation. They answer, "I am an accountant," "I am a welder," or "I am a pilot." The less they like their work, the more stress they will feel when they identify themselves in this way. The less successful they are at their work, the more guilt they will feel when they identify themselves with reference to it. In fact, some men tell me they feel as though they are borrowing an identity, rather than owning an

identity, because they do not deserve their occupational "titles."
Hal says:

> "I call myself an accountant, but I'm not really an accountant. I never
> even got certified. I kept thinking that I'd rather not be certified than fail
> the examination—so here I am. I push a pencil around numbers all
> day. I guess that makes me a clerk, but I don't like to call myself that.
> Soon the computers will put me out of accounting altogether. Then
> what will I be?"

Women, when they are asked to identify themselves, do not
usually refer to their occupation first. "Woman," "wife," or "mother" are statistically the more frequent first responses. The less
they like their work, the less identified they feel with it. Unlike
men, they do not often experience identity crises when they
experience job dissatisfaction, and they do not often experience
guilt when they think they are not performing well on the job.
On the contrary, women tell me that they experience guilt
when they have job *satisfaction* and when they *are* performing
well on the job because they are usually putting in extra time at
the office and preoccupied at home.

Perhaps the most fascinating difference between the ways
men and women view success is their explanation of their success. Whereas men feel that success is usually the result of hard
work, psychologist Madeline Hirschfeld found that women tend
to feel that success is more the result of luck than ability. Both
beliefs can, of course, lead to stress. If a man is not successful,
he is likely to blame himself for not working hard enough—
even when the problem is circumstantial rather than personal.
If a woman is successful, she is likely to feel that the achievement is precarious and can vanish overnight. Another way to
handle fear of failure or fear of success is to handicap yourself.
That is, start your projects late, overschedule yourself, and make
sure that your health is never what it should be. You have now
provided yourself with excuses in case you fear failure, or protection against the likelihood of reaching your goals in case you
fear success.

A better way to cope with goals, games, and guilt is to replace magical formulae and compulsive competitiveness with realistic appraisals of success opportunities and realistic appraisals of your own capabilities. Seek out information on the former, and ask for feedback on the latter. In Chapter 7, we will take a more detailed look at the stresses associated with work and striving for achievement.

"I DO'S" AND "I DON'TS"

Although the divorce rate is still high in the 1980s, the marriage and remarriage rates are also high for men. Married men live longer than single, divorced, or widowed men, and report more general life satisfaction, according to most surveys and reports. Why, then, did the majority of younger men responding to the Male Stress Survey list the decision to marry as one of the major stresses in their lives?

In her book *The Hearts of Men*, Barbara Ehrenreich points out that the young man today neither needs nor gets the same type of wife that his father did. Wives most often work full- or part-time now. They no longer reflect their husbands' status by caring for them and their children full-time. In fact, she suggests, the man's "liberation" from being the sole provider for his family has liberated him from the necessity for commitment. His sports car and his condo address provide status, instead. Dating becomes entertainment or sexual excitement, rather than a search for the "little woman."

If all this is true, then marriage becomes an option for men, not a social, economic, or sexual necessity. With an increased sense of choice comes an increased sense of hesitation and stress. "Since I don't really *have* to get married," a man thinks, "why do it?"

The answer for most men is that they have an *expectation of "primariness."* A man wants to be the most important person in someone's life. And that person is his wife!

Women, on the other hand, do not often expect primariness

from their husbands, although they would like it. They expect to share their man with his job, children, friends, and hobbies. They do, however, have *expectations of permanence*.

It is not that they are unaware of the high divorce rates and the decrease in social pressure to stay married. It is probably that women need their "expectations of permanence" to reduce their anxiety about starting a family. If they believed they would soon be running a single-parent household, their interest in motherhood might be seriously affected.

Once married, men and women again show stress differences. Men complain of *role confusion*; women complain of *role multiplication*. Role confusion for men is a relatively new phenomenon dating from the mid-1970s. Traditional husband and father roles had been unchanged for many, many generations. The modern male, however, is faced with mixed messages. He is still supposed to be strong, but he is now expected to be gentle as well. He is still expected to be a hard worker, but he is now expected to be unthreatened by his wife's work and help out with housework. He is still expected to assemble and paint the new crib, but now to change the diapers and feed the baby as well. For many men, it's simply not clear what a husband and father is supposed to be like today. Between the macho male at one extreme and the maternal male at the other, there is still a vast, uncharted territory.

As women try to combine housework, homework, and work-work, one would expect role confusion to plague them as much as it does men. But for women, the marital stress of the 1990s is role multiplication. Her roles are not changing—they are just piling up. The married woman of today knows that she is a wife, usually a job-holder, and often a mother. Her problem is not only that she expects herself to fill these three roles simultaneously, but that she also expects herself to do each on a full-time basis. She uses herself as cheap labor, adding more and more roles as the years go by. Soon she no longer has time for herself.

As men's roles continue to transform, however, they may very well end up a decade from now complaining of the very same thing! A study of married couples by sociologist Sarah Rosenfield, Ph.D., shows that when wives' earnings surpass their husbands', and when their jobs require a significant sharing of household chores, the men show signs of psychological stress, including higher levels of demoralization, depression, and anxiety—the very same problems of overload experienced by women today.

SHARING A WIFE, SHARING A LIFE

The male expectation of primariness, of being his wife's main concern, brings him into parenting with a stress handicap. As much as he loves his child, he must also admit to himself that he is no longer his wife's one-and-only. He is now sharing her time and attention—even her body—with their baby. Compounding this stress is the guilt he feels about any resentment he holds toward his wife or baby. Further compounding it is the reality that his mornings and nights will be different from now on!

His wife is not in a parallel position. She does not usually feel stressed because she must share her spouse with her child. Quite the contrary, her stress is often relieved when Daddy takes the baby for a while because so many mothers are going it alone. The extended family, the experienced grandmother, and the familiar family doctor usually are no longer around. The main issue for mothers is finding time to get away from all demands, even loving ones.

Men are expected to be caring, sharing, and involved with their children. But men are still also expected to be bread-winners and disciplinarians. Where are the role models for these fathers? From whom do they learn the ropes?

Not from women. Women are too busy trying to cope with too many roles themselves. If they want to move from working inside the home to working outside the home, they may not find many support systems available. If they choose full-time mothering as their career, they worry that they are not holding up their share of the family's economic burdens, nor developing their skills in case they become part of the divorce statistics. These women may become casualties of the "mommy wars"— an implicit (and sometimes explicit) rivalry between women who work inside the home and women who work outside the home—which only ends up making both sides feel guilty about the road not traveled! So neither fathers nor mothers escape special stresses in the nineties. We can only hope that the current changes in parental roles become clarified, and therefore more satisfying, to all concerned, so that we become balanced role models to the next generation of young parents.

DIVORCE DIFFERENCES

Next to the death of a spouse or child, divorce is probably the most stressful event of a man's (or woman's) life. The type of stress experienced depends on the type of divorce: hostile or friendly, equitable or financially lopsided, with or without a custody battle, coming after a few months or a few decades, mutual or unilateral.

The difference between male and female divorce stress is not actually the type of stress they have, but how stressed other people perceive them to be. Women who are left by their husbands are worried about; men who are left by their wives are treated with less concern:

"Wait until he gets out there—he'll love the single life!"
"He'll be grabbed up in no time."
"No problem. He can start again."

Since men have been raised to appear in control of their emotions and fear the loss of emotional control, they indeed seem to be less affected by their divorces than do women. Life and work go on, they seem to be saying. Actually, all the divorced men I surveyed missed daily contact with their children and regretted separation from them even if they were happy with the way their ex-wives mothered.

> "Listen to me. I've been going through the worst time of my life and nobody believes it. Everybody says, 'Hey, free at last.' Free at last. Guilty at last, yes. Sick at last, yes. Going crazy, yes. Not knowing what to do with myself, yes. Depressed, definitely. Thinking about my kids with another man, yes. Free? No."

Some fathers say that they dread "visiting days" with their children because they feel their children are, indeed, just visitors. "How should I entertain them?" "What should I buy them?" "What do they like to eat?" "How do they feel about these visits?" "Would they rather be with their friends?" How very different a feeling than that created by the old shout, "Hey, Dad's home!"

Discomfort is not for weekends only. Fathers call during the week, ask for their children, and get monosyllabic boys and girls who would rather be watching television. Fathers plan trips and surprises, and get only grunts or tired reminders that they had done the same thing last year with their scout troop. Fathers remind themselves that their children are probably better off with their mothers and each other than with themselves, and then try to convince themselves that it's true. Whereas women are stressed by having to head single-parent households, there are equally as many divorced fathers stressed by trying to parent from a distance.

SEX AND THE SEXES

Although more will be said in later chapters about the stresses of divorced men, the effect of stress on sex, and the stresses of aging, these factors are also being mentioned here to illustrate male/female stress differences. Sex stresses, for example, can be dramatically different for men than for women. Sex therapists describe the primary male sex stress as *performance anxiety;* the primary female sex stress I would call *preoccupation anxiety.*

A woman in this culture can be preoccupied and ambivalent about sex in various situations or with certain partners because she has been confronted all her life with contradictory messages:

- Be sexy and seductive, not sexual and assertive.
- Say "yes" if you want to please your man; say "no" if you want him to respect you.
- Maximize your pleasure by communicating your sexual requests; but minimize your partner's displeasure by avoiding putting sexual demands on him.
- Be sexually spontaneous; but guard against unwanted pregnancy.

A man in this culture can be plagued by performance anxiety in most situations and with many partners because he has been confronted all his mature life with the following messages:

- A man can't fake an orgasm.
- A man can't fake an erection.
- A man can't fake arousal.
- A man can't hide a "failure."

To add to a man's anxiety about performance, along come reports on the woman's capacity for multiple orgasm and the tapering of a man's virility after eighteen years of age! He may be able to court younger women, but can he satisfy them? he wonders. One bout of erectile problems, and he adds *anticipatory anxiety* to performance anxiety. One bout of premature ejaculation, and he also adds *control anxiety.* Chapter 3 will deal in more detail with sex and the Male Stress Syndrome.

GROWING OLD TOGETHER?

Both men and women age, of course, but for men there is usual-ly more to fear. Although women associate aging with loss of physical beauty, loss of social and sexual value, and loss of a spouse, aging for men is associated with death. Retirement may remind a man of his impending death, failing health may remind him, and dying friends may remind him. The more stressed he is over this, the more he is at high risk for male stress symptoms. Just look at the following facts:

- Prior to the age of sixty-five, men die from heart attacks at a rate of almost three to one as compared to women. After sixty-five, the rate is two to one.

- There are twice as many male deaths from accidents as female deaths.

- Men are four times more likely to commit suicide than women. An isolated elderly man is 1,350% more likely to commit suicide than a woman the same age.

- There are twice as many male deaths from liver disease as female deaths.

- There are ten times more male deaths than female deaths from HIV infection.

Life expectancy for males born in 1991 is seventy-two; for females it's seventy-nine. This seven-year gap in life expectancy is not uniform throughout life, however. It begins to narrow somewhat around age twenty and continues to decrease as men and women age. Still, at every point in life, women outlive men. Women who are sixty-five now can expect to live an average nineteen more years; men sixty-five, only fifteen more years. That means that at age sixty-five and older there are 8.5 million widows and only 1.9 million widowers, a ratio of about four women to every man—good news for single older men looking for partners!

But when a man begins to lose his health, his youth, or his

stamina, he becomes afraid that he has lost his ability to function. Functioning on the job, around the house, and in bed are vital to a masculine self-image. Men are "instrumental"—they make things happen. When they can't and their sense of control drops, their stress soars. Actually, some men responding to the Male Stress Survey said that they'd *prefer* to die quickly when young, rather than die slowly as they aged.

Many men are also aware that they will not survive as well without their wives as with them. The statistics emphasize this. Studies have shown that for older men whose wives have died, the mortality rate increases 48 percent—greater than that of men the same age who are still married—and a higher rate than women whose husbands have died. These men probably do not parent themselves as well as they should or as well as their wives did. Widows, then, may lose their relationship, their financial security, their sexual partner, and their social status when their spouses die—but widowers are more likely to lose their lives. However, if older widowers remarry soon after the death of their spouses—and most of them do—they better their chances of survival.

These are some of the most important stresses that contribute to the Male Stress Syndrome. In later chapters, we'll look at them in more detail and also discuss techniques to help counter or manage them. First, though, some background on the physical nature of stress, the symptoms it produces in a man's body, and the early warning signals that can help save your life.

2 GOOD STRESS, BAD STRESS, AND MALE STRESS

STRESS CAN BE DEFINED AS ANY DEMAND THAT REQUIRES ADJUSTMENT OR adaptation. Therefore, marriage, separation, divorce, and remarriage would each qualify as a stress. So too would a jet flight into a different time zone, a tennis game or a night at the bowling lanes, a promotion at work, a demotion at work, or a loss of work. Some of these stresses sound "bad," but some of them sound "good." Are they all equally damaging or dangerous? Absolutely not. Imagine this:

You are fourteen years old, out in center field, unaware of the hot sun beating down, and focused entirely on the pitcher and the batter. Every muscle in your body is ready for action. The pitcher lobs the ball, the batter swings, there's a blur of white where the ball leaves the bat, and in a fraction of a second you are running to meet it. Your heart is pumping twice as fast as normal, your blood pressure is high, and you are panting for breath. You take a quick look over your shoulder, make a split-second correction, and try a tremendous leap upward. The ball thunks into your glove and you run toward the infield, grinning.

Are you under stress? Imagine this:

You are forty years old and celebrating your fourteenth wedding anniversary. You and your wife are alone, with a bottle of wine, two flickering candles, and lots of love. She is massaging your back and you are remembering your honeymoon. Your memories become misty as the present brings more and more pleasure. You begin to focus all your attention on the touch of her hands and the sensations begin to arouse you. Your heart rate gradually increases until it is twice as fast as normal, your blood pressure is high, and you are breathing rapidly. You begin to make love to her.

Are you under stress? Imagine this:

It is Thursday night; you have been playing poker for three hours and your shirt is damp with perspiration. You're not hungry, but you are munching anyway while you wait for all the hands to fold, sure that tonight you will be the big winner. Your heart is beating rapidly, your energy is going strong, and your face is flushed. The stakes may be limited, but they are high and your cards look great. You feel as if you have been playing for days and would like to continue for weeks. You grunt when they ask what you've got, you groan when they demand your hand, and then you grin when you win.

Are you under stress?

Actually, you *are* under stress in each case—good stress. The body has mobilized for action by increasing heart rate, respiration, adrenaline output, perspiration, and muscle tension. And in each case you have taken action. The softball was caught, love was expressed, and the card game was won. The body's stress management system did exactly what it was designed to do— help you meet short-term demands for energy and action.

Good stress, then, creates a short-term feeling of exhilaration. Bad stress, on the other hand, creates long-term physical and psychological wear and tear. Imagine being unexpectedly fired from your job before you could quit. Imagine being forced to retire before you decided to leave. Imagine your son ill, your daughter injured, or your wife disabled with no assured recovery. Imagine your brother missing in action. Imagine a transfer that will take you away from your family. Imagine a transfer that will take your lover away from you. The vital difference between good stress and bad stress is determined by three factors:

1. *Your sense of choice.* If the demand is one you have chosen, it will feel more like "stimulation" than stress. In fact, many men are stimulus junkies. They choose to overschedule rather than underschedule themselves, and they work better under pressure. The key to "stimulation," though, is that the demand is chosen. If a demand is thrust on you instead, it will be experienced as stress.

2. *Your degree of control.* As your real or perceived control over a situation diminishes, your real and perceived stress increases. Compare, for example, being the passive passenger in a taxi with a pregnant wife in labor, stuck in the midst of midtown traffic, to being in the driver's seat in your own car, racing down the parkway to the county hospital. At least the driver can use up some adrenaline being active! It is difficult enough to give up control willingly—imagine how much stress increases if a demand requires that you give up control unwillingly or ambivalently.

3. *Your ability to anticipate consequences.* Adaptation and adjustment are most difficult when demands and outcomes are least predictable. The assembly-line operator always knows what is coming down the line next—he may be figuratively bored to death. The control-tower operator never knows what is coming next—he may be literally stressed to death.

Each of the imaginary "good stress" situations was entered into by choice. Each offered a degree of control. Each had limited and somewhat predictable consequences. Like the project you try to complete ahead of schedule, like the new customer you try to sign up, like the new design you want to restructure, like the speech you are going to deliver—each of these situations has a beginning and an end. And when it's over, it is usually definitely over. If you were successful, you feel tired but terrific. If you were not successful, you just feel tired.

What, however, would you feel if you were suddenly unemployed and needed lengthy retraining; demoted but stuck in the job; faced with the illness of your child, parent, or wife? What would you feel if you had no choice about a transfer, no control over your financial problems, or no way to predict the outcome of an illness? Bad stress.

When our stress management systems are overused and abused by long-term stress, physical and psychological symptoms of exhaustion begin to appear. If the abuse continues, permanent damage can result. It is important to understand how this happens.

HOW THE BODY COPES WITH STRESS

According to Hans Selye, who pioneered stress research over thirty years ago, the body copes with stress in three ways:

1. Stress messages travel from the brain through motor nerves to the "action" muscles in the arms, legs, and skeletal system, preparing them for sudden, explosive motion.

2. Stress messages travel from the brain through the autonomic nerves to vital organs, increasing heart rate, blood pressure, blood sugar levels, respiration, and red blood cell count. This, in turn, increases the supply of oxygen and energy available to the body. The same pathway also slows down intestinal movement, since digestion must yield to action in an emergency.

3. Stress messages travel from the brain to the adrenal gland and the hypothalamus. The adrenal gland regulates the release of adrenaline into the bloodstream as a fast-acting general stimulant. The hypothalamus, the "emotion center" of the brain, signals the pituitary and the adrenal cortex to release hormones into the bloodstream that offer slow-acting stress protection. The hor-

mones alter the salt/water balance of the blood to raise blood pressure; stimulate the release of thyroid hormones to speed up metabolism, allowing rapid conversion of food to energy; and raise the white blood cell count, affecting some immune and allergic responses.

These biochemical, cardiovascular, and muscle-tone changes prepare the body for either a "fight," "flight," or "fright" reaction, and they probably evolved at a time when stress meant an external and immediate threat. The "fight" response may have helped a man defend his territory or his mate. The "flight" response may have helped him escape from a wild animal. The "fright" response may have saved him from a natural disaster. In today's world, however, stress is too often internal rather than external, and chronic rather than intermittent. Instead of running from bears, we are running to buses and trains. Instead of fighting enemies, we are fighting anxieties. Instead of fearing avalanches, we are terrified of aging.

Actually, relaxation would be more helpful in these present-day stress situations than would the responses of increased heart rate, respiration, and blood pressure. But our stress management system reacts to being stuck in bumper-to-bumper traffic just as it would to a stress that requires action. Are we going to leave our car in the middle of the gridlocked intersection because our body is set for flight? Are we going to jump out of our car and beat up the motorist in front of us because our body is set for fight? Or are we going to sit in traffic and feel our heart working overtime, our digestion shutting down although we just gulped breakfast, and our muscles tensing for action that will never come?

Because our stress mobilization system is relatively non-specific, it will put our body through the same changes whether we get good news, bad news, or even no news. Dr. Selye called these physiological changes the General Adaptation Syndrome. If your stress is "good stress," under your control and short-term, your body will have a chance to rest after the General Adaptation Syndrome has been activated. But if your stress is long-term and beyond your control, your body will not have a chance to rest and you may begin to experience stress symptoms.

THE EFFECTS OF
SHORT- AND LONG-TERM STRESS

Stress symptoms are called *psychosomatic,* a term that literally means "mind-body." That is, psychological or "mind" stress is producing physiological or "body" effects. Sometimes extended stress produces wear and tear on healthy organs and systems. Sometimes it aggravates an already damaged or diseased weak link, such as an ulcerated stomach lining. Sometimes there is a predisposition toward a psychosomatic dysfunction, such as a heart defect, which emerges under stress. Sometimes stress diminishes defenses against disorders, diseases, and dysfunctions. Sometimes stress overwhelms healthful habits, as when it leaves us too tired to exercise. Sometimes it introduces unhealthful habits, as when we reach for a drink or a cigarette for a "quick fix."

Too often the term psychosomatic is misunderstood to mean "imaginary." Psychosomatic symptoms are *not* imaginary! Ulcers are real, asthma is real, and heart attacks are real. Think of psychosomatic illness this way: If you didn't know that your rapid heartbeat, tight stomach, shallow breathing, and flushed face were part of the stress response after a basketball game, you would conclude that you were sick. If these stress responses were to continue for too long, you *would* become sick.

Take respiration, for example. Under stress, breathing becomes more rapid—sometimes twice as fast as normal. If the stress is short-term stimulation, the additional oxygen injected into the bloodstream is used up and panting has served its purpose. If the stress is long-term, however, rapid respiration may continue until you have a dry mouth and irritated nasal passages, chest pains because the diaphragm muscles are cramping, and more. Rapid, shallow breathing not only increases the amount of oxygen in the bloodstream, it also decreases the amount of carbon dioxide in the bloodstream. Because it is high levels of carbon dioxide that trigger the breathing reflex, not low levels of oxygen, this decrease in the blood's carbon dioxide levels during stress signals the nervous system that fewer breaths are needed. Fewer breaths are indeed taken, and now you may begin to feel dizzy. You have hyperventilated by expelling carbon dioxide too quickly.

Hyperventilation can be managed by breathing into and out of a paper bag to return carbon dioxide to your lungs and raise its level in your bloodstream enough to trigger the breathing reflex. But other stress chain reactions may be far more difficult to remedy quickly. For example, under stress the large skeletal muscles are kept in a state of action readiness by a shift in blood flow toward those muscles and away from the skin and the gastrointestinal tract. First you may notice cold hands and cold feet, then your complexion may become pale or sallow, and finally you may begin to experience migraine headaches or high blood pressure.

Higher blood sugar levels, which are part of the stress reaction, also produce a chain of effects. First these sugar levels stimulate the release of additional insulin to break the sugars down. If too much insulin is produced, blood sugar levels fall too far, a condition known as hypoglycemia. The result is fatigue and a craving for "quick fixes," like the nicotine in cigarettes, the caffeine in coffee, or the sugars in candy. These, of course, stimulate even greater insulin production, and the low blood sugar cycle continues.

Another stress chain reaction affects the digestive system. Under stress, the rhythmic smooth muscle contractions necessary to push food through the stomach and intestine slow down, and gastric glands diminish their output. Soon gastritis, nausea, or constipation may develop. Eventually, the glucocorticoids—hormones produced under stress—indirectly increase stomach acidity, and with it heartburn and the risk of ulcers.

Actually, an excessive amount of glucocorticoids—or cortisol, in human beings—is emerging as the prime culprit in stress-related diseases. This steroid released by the adrenal gland is necessary to life—it's thanks to glucocorticoids that we can mobilize energy rapidly in order to fight or take flight. Glucocorticoids put off all our other bodily functions (digestion, reproduction, muscle repair, fighting infections, and so on) so that we can respond to the emergency that requires our immediate attention. Under normal conditions, our body turns those glucocorticoids on when it needs them, then turns them off when it doesn't. But if everything feels like an emergency, day after day, the flow of glucocorticoids is overstimulated until the system *can't* turn itself off and our normal bodily functions are disrupted. As a result, our immune system may be suppressed and there may even be organ damage, including death of neurons in the brain which control bodily functions. The bottom line is that excessive glucocorticoids accelerate aging.

PROBLEMS IN THE IMMUNE SYSTEM

The immune system is not a single system, but a variety of systems that work together in ways we still don't clearly comprehend. But we do know that stress harms at least some parts of the immune system. For example, Steven Schleifer and other researchers at Mount Sinai Medical Center in New York found that men whose wives had died of breast cancer showed a significant decrease in the activity levels of white blood cells, or leukocytes, which play a major role in defending the body against a variety of diseases. Schleifer thinks that stress-released hormones are responsible. Lack of sleep and strenuous exertion also reduce leukocyte activity, but in those cases it bounces back to normal in a day or so. Under stress, the effect can last for months.

Another immune system agent, salivary immunoglobulin (s-IgA), is also influenced by stress. Normally present in the mouth, s-IgA protects against bacterial and viral diseases, especially respiratory infections and dental cavities. Working with dental students, a team headed by psychologist John Jemmott of Princeton University saw the secretion of s-IgA decrease during stressful exam periods—especially among Type A students, who have a high drive for power and success. After the school term was over, their s-IgA levels fell even further. Dr. Jemmott thinks that this may be because they were brooding about their past performance, or because they had no chance to work off their stress during vacation.

Even susceptibility to the common cold may be stress-related. After all, the mucous membranes in the respiratory system become drier because of hyperventilation and, therefore, more irritable and less protected against bacteria and viruses. Cortisone levels are down and inflammations are up. Temperature regulation is altered, and the immune system is consequently affected. Does this mean that an extended visit from your in-laws might really be the cause of your cold? Could be! Does it mean that stress symptoms should be taken seriously? Definitely!

MALE STRESS

Far too often men ignore stress symptoms, denying their potential consequences and avoiding having to address their causes. When women who participated in the Male Stress Survey were asked to check the physical signs of stress they noticed in their men—husbands, fathers, or sons—they most frequently said they saw the following (from a total list of twenty-six items):

insomnia
headaches

allergies (hives, hay fever, and congestion)
teeth grinding, jaw clenching (temporomandibular joint
     muscle spasms, or TMJ)
nausea, indigestion, and heartburn
backaches and stiff necks

When men themselves were asked about their physical symptoms of stress, one of the few symptoms they consistently reported noticing was that they perspired more under stress! What about all the symptoms reported by the women? Men acknowledge them, but do not usually attribute them to stress; they tend to attribute them simply to age. Their reports of physical problems from the Male Stress Survey can be tabulated according to age approximately like this:

Symptoms	Ages			
	18-29	30-39	40-49	50+
high blood pressure				X
muscle aches			X	X
gastritis/ulcers			X	X
heartburn		X	X	X
headache	X	X	X	X

According to this information, men seem to add new stress symptoms to their old ones as they age. If—as many do—they think each is a sign of a malignancy or premature aging rather than stress, their fears will compound their stresses and multiply their symptoms. If they are avoiding medical check-ups as well, more serious stress-related disorders may develop.

Check yourself on the summary of *general* stress symptoms below. (For the women reading this, see how many of these symptoms are true for your husband, lover, father, or sons.)

_____ irritable bowel syndrome
_____ swallowing problems (esophageal spasms)
_____ hyperventilation

_____ asthma
_____ rheumatoid arthritis
_____ allergies
_____ skin disorders
_____ heartburn (hyperacidity)
_____ neck aches or backaches
_____ cold sweats
_____ anxiety attacks
_____ constipation or diarrhea
_____ chest pains
_____ dizziness
_____ chronic fatigue
_____ headaches
_____ insomnia

You need not begin to add up the check marks. If you or a man in your life has even *one* check on this list, then stress is probably involved. Even those disorders on the list that might not be caused by stress can certainly be aggravated by stress.

In addition to the more general stress symptoms, which are shared by women under stress, men under stress show some symptoms that are uniquely theirs, more frequently theirs, or more dangerous when they are theirs. These symptoms are:

> hypertension (high blood pressure)
> atherosclerosis (high cholesterol level)
> heart attack (myocardial infarction)
> heart failure
> peptic ulcer (gastric or duodenal)
> alcoholism
> erectile dysfunction
> premature ejaculation
> retarded ejaculation

Some of these ailments and disorders relate to the male physiology. Some reflect social, sexual, and psychological demands associated with being a man in this culture. Some are affected by early upbringing and developmental history. Some reflect life-style. And some are brought on by the life changes and events that are part of a man's experience.

In the chapters that follow, we'll be examining how all these physical, social, and psychological factors affect your stress responses and your health. The most important point to remember is that male stress symptoms cannot be ignored. Even those traditionally male symptoms that are being seen more frequently among women—such as nicotine addiction, alcoholism, heart disease, high blood pressure, and angina—seem to show their effects on men at an earlier age. Understanding how stress affects the body in general, and the male body in particular, is vital for improving both the quality of your life and the *length* of it.

3 STRESS AND THE MALE BODY

Are men the stronger sex? In physical size and muscle mass, perhaps, but not when it comes to stress endurance. Although more men than women are conceived and born, by the end of one year the male/female ratio is reversed. More male fetuses die during their mothers' pregnancies, and more males die at birth and as newborns. Furthermore, as noted in Chapter 1, women live longer; there is an average life expectancy of seventy-nine years for girl babies and seventy-two years for boy babies. From birth to old age, then, men seem to die more easily than women.

In between these milestones, men don't seem to do as well either. They tend to lose the use of their legs and hands earlier, turn gray faster, experience hearing and eyesight loss sooner, and have memory problems at earlier ages. And as far as sex is concerned, the man's capacity to perform (though not his fertility) diminishes with age more sharply than the woman's capacity.

There are still other areas of male vulnerability. Men may be less sensitive to pain, and so they may be less aware of physical problems until symptoms are serious. They are also more apt to minimize or deny their pain, causing them to seek treatment much later in the disease process. According to the Men's Health Network, a Washington, D.C.-based advocacy group, men are three times less likely to visit a physician than are women. Although they have greater physical strength, they have a lower fat/muscle ratio, and thus fewer energy reserves. Since males, even from birth, seem to react less to touch than females, it is possible that they are less easily soothed and comforted when they are stressed.

Do men have any stress *advantages* to balance these stress handicaps? Research suggests that they probably have two built-in advantages in dealing with short-term emergencies and temporary stress:

1. According to Karl Pribam, at the University of California at Santa Cruz, young boys show greater right-brain dominance than girls. The right hemisphere of the brain deals with nonverbal, symbolic, spontaneous responses to information, whereas the left hemisphere governs language, logic, and labels. In other words, during their early years, when they are learning to deal with the world, boys may be predisposed to evaluate and react to situations *immediately* and *directly*. They may be ready to fight or flee, swing or fling or yell, while little girls are reacting to their world in a verbal, step-by-step fashion. This young male response very likely had a great survival value if you think of early mankind. Life in those days probably depended on fast action, not fast talk. Since boys seem to gain left-hemisphere dominance by high school years, control over these impulses is usually achieved. But male action impulses and responses are likely to remain as valuable stress advantages in emergencies.

2. The male hormone testosterone is associated with rough-and-tumble play, extraversion, high activity levels, and assertiveness. Equally interesting is the suggestion of John Bancroft, reported in *The Clinics of Obstetrics and Gynecology*, that men with low testos-

terone levels can more easily be distracted. In short, testosterone may heighten the ability to focus and stay focused on a situation. This would be an important survival capability for early man trying to exist in a physically dangerous world, or for today's man trying to concentrate in a noisy, polluted world.

Adding together both the good and bad news about male stress management, it is possible to see a *stress responsiveness* that is activated in emergency situations. That is, it may be that since young men seem to react to stress nonverbally, rapidly, and with action; since they can focus and stay focused on high-arousal situations with great intensity; and since they develop more physical strength and can be less aware of low-level pain sensations than women, they are primed and equipped to handle immediate action demands.

What happens to the male body, however, when the stress goes on and on? Disorders, diseases, dysfunctions, and, often, death.

What follows in this chapter is the real nuts-and-bolts information about how stress may be affecting you physically. These are the stress symptoms that can kill you, or severely compromise the quality of your life. (If you are not having such a great day, you might want to skip this section until tomorrow!) While this is vitally important information, it's not all so grim: in later chapters I'll be telling you about the early warning signs of stress that can help save your life, and teaching you stress management techniques that make living with the Male Stress Syndrome much easier.

THE RISK OF CARDIOVASCULAR DISORDERS

Cardiovascular disorders include disorders of the heart (cardio) and the blood vessels (vascular). Although we often refer to cancer as the most dreaded disease, there are almost twice as many deaths from cardiovascular diseases as there are cancer deaths. Almost one half of all deaths in this country are due to cardiovascular disorders.

For men, heart disease becomes the leading cause of death by approximately age forty, whereas for women this isn't the case until around age seventy. The coronary heart disease symptoms typically appear ten years earlier in men than in women, and first heart attacks for men occur twenty years earlier than for women. In fact, under age sixty-five, men are three times more likely than women to die of coronary heart disease. For all ages, heart disease rates and cardiovascular disease death rates (which include stroke) are more than twice as high in men as in women.

The reason the risk ratio begins to even out and then increase for women after sixty-five years is probably due to hormonal changes. Androgens, the male sex hormones, seem to increase blood cholesterol while estrogens, the female sex hormones, seem to decrease blood cholesterol. With decreases in testosterone, therefore, a man's cardiovascular morbidity and risk may improve, while the protective effect of estrogens on women may decline with menopause.

Of the many cardiovascular diseases, disorders, and dysfunctions, four are particularly associated with long-term stress in men: hypertension, atherosclerosis, heart attack, and heart failure. Each may also reflect a genetic predisposition, aneurysm (a weakness in the blood vessel wall), or damage, but the stress link is usually there, too. In fact, decades of research on the relationship between stress and cardiovascular disease have convinced the American Heart Association that stress is a secondary coronary risk factor, interacting with the primary risk factors of hypertension (high blood pressure), high serum cholesterol, diabetes, and smoking.

HYPERTENSION

Hypertension refers to chronic high blood pressure. Blood pressure rises if the heart rate increases or the arterial blood vessels constrict. Short-term this adjustment can be useful; long-term it can be perilous. Heart contractions in the average man occur about seventy times per minute, about forty million times a year, and pump more than 2,000 gallons of blood a day. During exercise, sexual arousal, or stress, the number of heart contractions per minute can double. This will double the strain on the heart muscle and the arteries. Since neither exercise nor sexual arousal can go on forever, this type of increase in blood pressure creates no danger unless a cardiovascular problem already exists. Since stress arousal *can* go on and on, anxiety and aggravation can be dangerous.

One danger associated with chronic high blood pressure is that of heart enlargement. To continue supplying blood to the body through constricted or narrowed arteries, the heart has to work harder than it was designed to work. To maintain the required blood flow against this resistance, the heart muscle typically enlarges, although its own supply of blood may not proportionally increase at the same rate. Thus, the heart is doing more work, receiving fewer nutrients, and building up more waste products. Soon it will tire like any other muscle, spasm painfully (angina pectoris), and maybe even fail.

A second danger is that increased blood pressure can burst an artery or push a blood clot or mass of foreign material into a small vessel. The clot is called a thrombus, and thrombosis is the process by which the clot forms. Similarly, an embolus is the mass of foreign material and an embolism is the process of blocking the vessel. If the rupture, embolus or thrombus, deprives tissue of blood supply, it will die (infarct). When the tissue affected is brain tissue, the condition is called a cerebrovascular accident, or a "stroke." Depending upon which area of the brain is damaged, the symptoms might be a loss of speech, loss of muscle control, loss of consciousness, or even loss of life. When the tissue affected is heart muscle, the condition is called a myocardial (heart muscle) infarction, or "heart attack." If too much heart muscle dies or is replaced by tough scar tissue, if too little blood supply can be rerouted to the heart muscle, or if too many of the nerves that regulate the heartbeat are impaired, cardiac arrest may result.

ATHEROSCLEROSIS

Atherosclerosis is the process by which fatty deposits (atheroma) accumulate and build up on the inner lining of the arteries. Fats dissolved in the blood, such as cholesterol, may be precipitated out of solution faster in the presence of prolonged elevated blood pressure.

Arteriosclerosis, on the other hand, is the hardening of the walls of the arteries themselves, making them less elastic and less able to endure and perhaps cushion the higher systolic pressures generated by the heart (the pressure generated as the heart pumps blood into the arterial system).

The greater the duration of stress, the longer the increase in blood pressure. The longer the increase in blood pressure, the greater the amount of fatty deposits. It is not clear whether the high blood pressure results from the reduced inner diameter of the arteries, or whether the high blood pressure forces the deposits onto the inner walls of the arteries, or both. What *is* clear is that there is a connection between stress, high blood pressure, and atherosclerosis. It is the *cholesterol connection*.

A large part of the waxy, fatty atheroma that can coat the arteries' walls in atherosclerosis is cholesterol. Cholesterol is used throughout the body for mending membranes and producing certain secretions. Although cholesterol is ingested when we eat egg yolks, dairy products, and animal fats, most of the cholesterol found circulating in the bloodstream is probably manufactured in the liver. While the cholesterol is circulating in solution, it poses no problem. Once it is deposited on arterial walls, blood clots can cling to it and create a thrombus that may block the artery entirely, or break off (embolize) and block a smaller, more peripheral arteriole.

Researchers currently suspect that stress encourages the buildup of cholesterol deposits in two ways:

1. Vincent DeQuattro of the University of Southern

California Medical Center at Los Angeles found that patients with high blood pressure had more noradrenaline in their bodies than subjects with lower blood pressure. Noradrenaline, a neurotransmitter secreted as part of the stress chain reaction, constricts blood vessels, thus raising blood pressure. It also remains in the bloodstream even after the stress situation is eliminated. If the stress situation is not eliminated, but continues long-term, or if the stress situations follow each other rapidly, the noradrenaline can remain in the bloodstream indefinitely—a permanent trigger for high blood pressure. High blood pressure, in turn, may be involved in nailing cholesterol into place—the wrong place.

2. Under stress, not only does blood pressure go up, but so may the amount of cholesterol in the blood. It seems that any type of stress, physical or psychological trauma, causes the adrenal cortex to secrete cortisol, which results in the mobilization of fatty acids. These fatty acids pour into the bloodstream and are metabolized by muscles in fight or flight situations, but are left circulating when there is more anxiety than action. Eventually, the fatty acids may convert to cholesterol deposits. Again, stress is implicated in the development of high blood pressure and atherosclerosis.

As blood flow dwindles and cholesterol count climbs, a man's anxiety about his health and heart risk are added to the stresses that helped to produce the condition in the first place. He can change his eating habits to reduce cholesterol intake. He can reduce the intake of animal (saturated) fats, which seem to facilitate the liver's production of cholesterol precursors. He can reduce his intake of highly unsaturated fatty acids, which often helps to decrease serum (blood) cholesterol somewhat. He can increase his exercise in order to "use up" the noradrenaline and epinephrine and the fatty acids that pour into the bloodstream during stress. He can take medication to lower his blood pressure or medication to tranquilize himself. But he can't stop the aging process and vascular changes that seem to go along with it.

HEART ATTACK/HEART FAILURE

Cardiovascular problems begin to appear in men by fifteen to twenty years of age. Why men have a twenty-year head start on cardiovascular problems compared to women is still something of a mystery, but as I noted it is suspected that hormonal differences mitigate these problems in most women until after menopause. This year, for example, it can be estimated that almost eight men out of every one hundred will die from heart problems, compared to only four women out of one hundred.

BEHAVIORAL FACTORS AND THE HEART

The man's vulnerability to heart attacks and heart failure cannot be blamed entirely on his physiology. His psychology has been clearly implicated by a decade of research. On the simplest level, stress changes not only neurotransmitters, secretions, and muscle tone, but it also changes *behavior*. Men under stress may eat more poorly, smoke more frequently, drink more alcohol, fall asleep later, or awake much earlier. These stress symptoms are behaviors which, of course, become stressors themselves. They represent attempts at coping that *don't work!* The cigarettes, alcohol, or food will not change an unemployment, divorce, or deadline problem. They reduce the sensations of stress for the moment, not the causes of stress in the long run.

Eric had bought the snack bar concession at the municipal community swimming pool, although he was neither a restaurateur nor a businessman—he was a pharmacist. He thought it would be lucrative and challenging. It soon became overwhelming, instead. He had equipment that kept breaking down, teenage cooks who kept quitting, rainy days that kept the customers home, and spoilage. He even found himself embroiled in a parents' committee action against "junk food." Eric began to smoke, again. He hadn't smoked in four years. When he wasn't reaching for a cigarette, he'd reach for the candy he sold to sweeten his day and boost his energy. The sugar highs were followed by sugar lows, which he'd try to counteract with a cup of coffee. At night he'd unwind with a few beers. The beers at night and aggravation all day had him asleep in front of the television by eight-thirty. By the end of the summer, he had gained almost fifteen pounds, was smoking a pack of cigarettes a day, and had dropped his regular exercise routine. His snack bar broke even; Eric did not!

Although many researchers have been forging stronger and stronger links between vascular problems and stress, one of the earliest reports is still the most famous. In 1974, when Meyer Friedman and Ray Rosenman wrote *Type A Behavior and Your Heart*, their conclusions worried a lot of men, and with good reason. Friedman and Rosenman found a significant correlation between achievement-oriented, competitive behaviors in men and a risk of cardiovascular disease. They suggested that the same characteristics that lead men to career success may be leading them to heart attacks!

Research over the years since then has attempted to pinpoint exactly which attributes of the Type A personality are really associated with increased risk of cardiovascular problems. Redford Williams, M.D., Director of Behavioral Research at Duke University Medical Center, and other researchers now believe that it's the anger, hostility, and cynical mistrust of others that contribute most heavily to heart attack risk. But all type A behaviors can increase stress levels, stress symptoms, and stress "fallout" for others.

What is the Type A male like? Chapter 7 will discuss Type A behaviors within the working world, but here is a general outline:

Competitiveness

Open about it or embarrassed by it, the Type A male is competitive. Some are motivated by the thrill of victory. Some are trying to avoid the agony of defeat. Some compete actively, making their challenge public. Some are closet competitors, upping their own quotas for themselves continually. Some compete all day, in every way—while driving, working, or playing. Some compete selectively, choosing specific battles or special opponents.

> Don doesn't describe himself as competitive since he takes orders well and likes being a team player. He is aware of being vigilant of others' accomplishments, but only, he claims, to prove to himself that he is as good as the next guy—not better. Most of his waking energy, in fact, is spent trying to be as good as the next guy. "That's a lot of energy," notes his wife.

Impatience

Type A men hate to wait. They would rather be late, and usually are. Waiting time may mean time for depressing or anxiety-provoking thoughts to intrude. Waiting time may mean money lost. Waiting time may result in feeling demeaned. True Type A's can't even wait for others to finish speaking, and complete their sentences for them. Sound familiar?

> Nat was twenty minutes early for his dental appointment. He felt relaxed and in control of his morning. Time for a quick stop to pick up a newspaper, he thought. While he was in the candy store, he started browsing for a paperback. "I can read in the waiting room," he thought. He paused to buy a lottery ticket at the checkout counter and then walked to the dentist's office down the block. By now he had used up nineteen minutes and the office building's elevator was out. He had to walk up six flights, was five minutes late, and had lost his sense of control over his morning. He had, however, avoided waiting for his appointment. Although he was unaware that he hated to wait, he had consistently been late for his dental appointments, tennis games, and car pool for seven years running.

Perfectionism

Type A's try to function so well that they need never be criticized. So why shouldn't everyone else try to be perfect also? Type A men are as much plagued by others' shortcomings as by their own. Their impatience and competitiveness combine with perfectionism to drive them to perform, perform, perform. They will do tasks themselves rather than delegate responsibility in order to make sure the tasks are done right. Even if they do pass the task to another, they will monitor its completion with the same energy—if not more—as if they had done it themselves. Being the child or wife of a Type A man is as difficult as being the Type A man himself!

> Mel was known as the "Memo King." He would give junior account executives assignments and then issue reams of follow-up instructions. He'd schedule more meetings with his assistants than he would if he were handling the client himself. He would also get a headache every day by noon. His assistant claimed he gave himself headaches trying to make sure his clients were spared them.

Polyphasic Behavior

This is perhaps the easiest Type A behavior to spot, and it consists of doubling and tripling up on activities simultaneously. If you scan the newspaper, sip your coffee, set up your desktop for the day, *and* take a telephone call from your first customer all at the same time, then you are definitely a Type A personality. Not only are you putting extra demands on your concentration, digestion, and energy, but you are depriving yourself of opportunities to relax while sipping coffee, *or* reading the newspaper, *or* setting up your desk. A polyphasic is suffering from what Dr. Friedman calls the "hurry sickness."

> Although Ian enjoyed board games, it was weeks since his son had set up the elaborate military grid that Ian had bought for him. They were going to play every night and keep a running score of their strategy points, but every night Ian would bring case folders to the table with him and find something inside that had to be taken care of immediately by telephone or by a file search in his home office. He'd try to take care of business when it was his son's turn at the game, but needed too much briefing every time he returned to continue the play. He was teaching his son that time together was a waste of his time. That was not his objective!

Hostility

Of all the Type A behaviors, it's chronic anger that research indicates is most dangerous. It's secret anger that can drive blood pressure up, and, remember, the risk of heart attack with it. For example, males ages eighteen to twenty-six who scored either high or low on a hostility scale were recruited for a study that measured blood pressure while the men tried to solve puzzles. The more hostile men had significantly higher blood pressure (BP) readings and poorer recovery to normal BP than less hostile men. Their BP was even higher when the laboratory technicians purposely harassed them (Suarez & Williams). And even young boys, ages six to eighteen, who are in families that show a lot of anger, aggression, and conflict were found to have a higher lipid ratio (too much "bad" cholesterol, not enough "good" cholesterol) than boys in more supportive families.

Feeling hostile and cynical, the Type A man sets up a negative self-fulfilling prophecy for his work and play relationships. He often expects the same competitiveness and impatience that he feels—and therefore gets it!

> Gordon had been at the same job for fifteen years but didn't count even one of his post office co-workers as his friend. He knew that he used to resent being supervised by Frank, and he assumed that the workers likewise resented being supervised by him now that Frank had retired. He knew that he used to laugh at the new guys when he was still working on the "floor level," and he assumed that the floor workers still did. He felt self-protective, acted aloof, and was treated like someone who didn't belong. He didn't want to belong, he told himself. And got angrier each year.

Actually the Type A man finds stress in every situation; and if it is not inherently there, he makes it stressful himself. He has turned his life over to long-term stress, and it is killing him. The link between cardiovascular problems and stress shows up in study after study:

- British researchers gave two puzzles and a deadline to twenty middle-aged men. They gave the same puzzle to twenty others, but let these men work at their own pace. Those under deadline pressure saw their blood pressures rise twice as high as those who were self-paced (Steptoe et al.).

- Chronic exposure to high noise levels at work consti- tute a stressor for Type A men. An Israeli study showed that Type A's respond to noise stress with higher levels of tension, blood pressure, and heart rate than type B's (Melamed et al.).

- First-year medical students were tested for mood states, perception of work pressure, and cardiovascular func- tion during both an exam week and a week in which no exams were given. There were increases in reports of anxiety, depression, and hostility, as well as greater heart rate measurement during the exam week, with Type A's showing greater increases in cardiovascular responses in not only the more stressful exam week but also during the week in which no exams were given (Lovallo et al.).

The bad news is that you need only *one of* the characteristics outlined above to be considered Type A. The good news is that simple changes such as learning to move, talk, and eat more slowly, as well as more complicated behavior modification such as developing patience and a positive perspective, *can* lower your risk of heart attack.

Long-range studies at Mt. Zion Hospital and Medical Center in San Francisco and at Stanford University School of Education now indicate that the stress-related risk of heart problems can, however, be reduced. For example, after almost five years, post-coronary subjects who altered their diets, exercised, and received counseling to reduce their Type A behavior and raise their self-esteem had *less than half* as many second heart attacks as subjects who received no counseling. According to cardiologist Meyer Friedman, the study director, and Carl Thorsen of Stanford University, only 12.9 percent of over 500 cardiac patients in the experimental group had a second heart attack, compared to 21 percent of the group who received diet and exercise advice only, and almost 32 percent of the subjects who dropped out of the study altogether. We'll look again at Type A behavior and how to cope with it in later chapters.

THE RISK OF ULCERS

Not all Male Stress Syndrome disorders, dysfunctions, or diseases are likely to be as fatal as cardiovascular problems. Gastrointestinal ulcers, for example, are usually thought of as more uncomfortable than life-threatening. Indeed, they are often unrecognized, ignored, or untreated for years. Eventually, however, ulcers can erode the stomach or intestinal wall and cause bleeding first, and then death. Approximately 6,000 deaths occur per year in this country due to ulcers, most of them men.

Gastric (stomach) or duodenal (intestinal) ulcers seem to develop when the protective mucinoid lining in an area is destroyed by digestive juices containing hydrochloric acid, to the point that it does not regenerate. Sheldon Lachman, author of *Psychosomatic Disorders: A Behavioristic Interpretation*, describes the ulcer as the result of "the gastrointestinal tract digesting itself."

How does stress result in this version of "eating yourself up alive"? Scientists hypothesize that many or all of the following factors may be interacting:

1. During stress, gastrointestinal peristalsis (rhythmic movement) becomes disturbed and the gastrointestinal lining may become abraded, "buckled," or even "broken." Once this happens, the hydrochloric acid can erode the wall behind the lining.

2. During stress, there can be an increase in gastric acidity which may ulcerate even a normal, intact mucinoid lining.

3. During stress, the stomach lining may become engorged with blood, possibly making it more vulnerable to bleeding.

4. During stress, the immune systems seem to be suppressed and healing slowed, while the opportunities for infection increase.

Almost 90 percent of all ulcers are duodenal (intestinal), painful, and a man's symptom. They can begin in men as young as twenty years old and are more likely to occur if he drinks alcohol excessively, eats rich or irritating foods, suffers from heartburn or stomach infections frequently, is genetically predisposed, is a Type A personality, and/or is experiencing long-term stress. If he smokes cigarettes, his risk of gastric ulcers may be up to five times greater than a nonsmoker's risk, and his risk of duodenal ulcer doubles. Furthermore, smoking seems to hinder healing once ulcers do occur. Women showing the same high-risk factors, however, are not likely to develop ulcers until after menopause. It is possible that the hormones responsible for premenstrual symptoms, postpartum depression, and menopausal problems are *protecting* women from ulcers and many types of cardiovascular problems.

As with all male stress symptoms, prevention is the best medicine. If an ulcer has already developed, x-rays can confirm the diagnosis. Then rest, a controlled diet, medication, including antibiotics, and stress management techniques such as those discussed in Chapter 9 are prescribed. Even when ulcers are not life-threatening, they are expensive. Dr. Lachman estimates that the national cost of ulcers due to disability payments, lost income, and medical expenses probably nears a billion dollars a year.

THE RISK OF ALCOHOLISM

According to the *Eighth Special Report of the U.S. Congress on Alcohol and Health,* of men who drink, 44 percent are classified as light drinkers, 37 percent are moderate drinkers, and 19 percent are heavy drinkers, compared to 7 percent of women who are heavy drinkers. High prevalence of heavier drinking among men was observed particularly among unemployed, divorced, separated, or widowed men, and among those with low incomes.

If you're wondering about the criteria for alcohol abuse, dependence, or both (see *Diagnostic and Statistical Manual of Mental Disorders*), at least three of the following criteria are required to diagnose alcohol dependence:

- Need for increased amounts of alcohol to achieve intoxication.
- Alcohol taken to relieve or avoid withdrawal symptoms.
- Inability to control the quantity of alcohol consumed.
- Neglect of important social and occupational activities.
- Drinking when it is physically hazardous.
- Continued drinking despite knowledge of having a problem.
- Legal problems.
- A great deal of time spent in activities to obtain alcohol, to drink, etc.
- These symptoms have occurred repeatedly over time.

As with other male stress symptoms, alcoholism is overdetermined—that is, it will take *many* factors interacting to produce the problem. New evidence suggests alcoholics may be metabolizing alcohol differently than nonalcoholics and must, for physical reasons, avoid alcohol for life. Other studies show a familial pattern to alcoholism that suggests either a genetic metabolic component or a learned response to stress. Obviously, the acceptability and availability of alcohol as a stress solution is of great importance, as well.

The irony is that alcohol doesn't really work as a stress solution. If you are drinking to "forget," you will find that alcohol will *improve* your memory for events and feelings *preceding* intoxication. Sobering up will therefore leave you feeling as bad as, if not worse than, you did before you drank. If you are drinking to get your feelings out, you are likely to feel guilty when you sober up. If you are drinking to distract yourself, you will instead have your bad mood exaggerated by alcohol. Just as drinking when you feel good makes you feel even "higher," drinking when you feel bad will make you feel worse.

What you really need if you or someone you love is an alcoholic is professional help to learn alternative stress management techniques, increase self-confidence, provide honest feedback, and manage withdrawal medically. Prevention and maintenance come from Male Stress Syndrome awareness.

THE RISK OF SEXUAL DYSFUNCTIONS

Which of the following statements are true and which are false?

_____ Sex can reduce stress symptoms.
_____ Stress can reduce sexual arousal.
_____ Morning erections mean a full bladder.
_____ Distracting yourself can slow down premature ejaculations.
_____ Alcohol enhances sexual performance.
_____ Impotence can be the result of too much masturbation.
_____ Most men with erectile problems have an androgen (testosterone) deficiency.

The first two statements are true. Sexual arousal can indeed reduce stress symptoms. Psychologically, sexual intimacy is a reminder that you are not alone in the world, that you have much to give; it can distract you from your short- and long-term stresses, can provide you with play and pleasure, can provide an opportunity for spontaneity and fantasy, and can leave you with a sense of lingering love, close comfort, sensual sleepiness, and/or renewed energy. Physically, sexual arousal, foreplay, and orgasm can use up the adrenaline (norepinephrine) that has been released into your bloodstream during stress; they can increase endorphin levels, which will give you a natural "high"; and they can even stimulate cortisone production, which will reduce allergic reaction and some types of arthritic inflammations.

Unfortunately, it works the other way around as well—stress

can reduce sexual arousal, your capacity for sex. This stress-sex link is rarely physiological, however. According to endocrinologist John Bancroft, as long as men have testosterone levels in the normal range (and most men with sexual dysfunction do), hormone treatment has little or no effect on erectile problems. Sex therapy focusing on reducing performance anxiety, fear of failure, couple and marital stress or conflicts, and misinformation, on the other hand, usually produces dramatic success.

All the remaining statements in the quiz on page 49 are *false:*

- Morning erections are thought to reflect the body's circadian (daily) rhythms, perhaps a rise in testosterone level that occurs in the early morning hours or a change in blood flow patterns. They are a sign that the genitals and hormone levels are physiologically normal and, although these erections diminish during urination, they are not *caused* by the need to urinate.

- Distracting yourself with baseball scores or stress-provoking preoccupations only permits an orgasm to "sneak up" on you more quickly if you have a tendency toward premature ejaculation. Sex therapy encourages paying *more* attention to sensations, not less.

- Alcohol, unfortunately, both giveth and taketh away sexually. By disinhibiting sexual impulses, it may fan the flames of desire. But by interfering with erectile capacity, it may wash away any chance of intercourse. Even worse, a man who is unfamiliar with this effect of alcohol might become so preoccupied with his potency after an alcohol-related "failure" that future attempts at lovemaking become sabotaged by his own fears. A vicious cycle is set in motion.

- Masturbation at any age is normal. In utero, male fetuses have spontaneous erections visible in sonograms. Single men in their thirties achieve at least 25 percent of their orgasms through masturbation. Ninety percent of men in their fifties report masturbation experiences. Semen is regenerated as it is expelled; the refractory period (erection loss) after ejaculation assures "rest" time, so there is no danger of becoming impotent. Masturbation can, however, be a male stress symptom if it is used to reduce *any* or *all* tensions, rather than sexual tension. If masturbation is used to reduce the tension of boredom, anger, disappointment, loss, anxiety, fear, loneliness, and work pressure, it is probably at that point an act of compulsion rather than one of pleasure.

- As I've noted, most men with sexual dysfunction have testosterone levels in the normal range, and hormone treatment has been found to have little or no effect on erectile problems.

ERECTILE DYSFUNCTION

Although the word "impotence," meaning powerlessness, has been replaced by the term "erectile dysfunction," most men who experience this stress symptom indeed report feeling powerless.

Tom is fifty-five years old and his wife is telling him not to worry. He has lost his erection again—and she's telling him not to worry. "I'm not worried," he says quietly. Not worried. Not worried about turning fifty-five the day before yesterday. Not worried about being impotent. She can fake sex and it makes no difference. But in his world his erection *does* make a difference, a big difference. There is a tingle in his fingertips, his stomach feels tight, and he is beginning to get a headache. Stay calm. Say it again. "I'm not worried," he says, and rolls onto his back, his heart beating too quickly.

Trouble achieving or maintaining an erection may mean no more than fatigue, too much alcohol, a medication side-effect, performance anxiety with a new partner, or prolonged anger at an old partner. If it occurs only at certain times, it is called "situational." If it occurs only with particular people, it is called "selective." If it occurs at all, it is likely to cause as much stress as the stress that produced it.

Many cases of stress-induced impotence, if left alone, would cure themselves. Typically, however, after only a very few episodes (sometimes all it takes is one) the man begins to worry about it. This adds to his stress—and his potency problems. Then he begins checking up on himself during foreplay to see how he's doing, and this makes having an erection almost impossible.

You should know that many medications and drugs that are used for stress symptoms or stress relief have possible adverse effects on sexual functioning. Psychiatrist Philip Luloff provides the following list of drugs that may lower libido and/or create some erectile problems. Ask your physician for more information if you are having a problem.

Heart and blood pressure drugs:	Atenolol (Tenormin)
	Propranolol (Inderal)
	Digoxin
	Dyazide
	Reserpine
Mood-management drugs:	Amitriptyline (Elavil)
	Chlorpromazine (Thorazine)
	Diazepam (Valium)
	Doxepin (Sinequan)
	Haloperidol (Haldol)
	Imipramine (Tofranil)
	Lithium
	Thioridazine (Mellaril)
Gastrointestinal drugs:	Chlordiazepoxide (Librax)
	Cimetidine (Tagamet)
	Dicyclomine Hydrochloride (Bentyl)
Mood-altering or "recreational" drugs:	Alcohol—erectile dysfunction
	Amphetamines—erectile dysfunction
	Cocaine—libido decrease

Heroin—libido decrease
and erectile dysfunction
Marijuana—libido decrease and
erectile dysfunction
Tobacco

According to the 1992 National Institutes of Health Consensus Development Conference on impotence, as many as thirty million men in the U.S. have full or partial erectile dysfunction. While erectile dysfunction in most men is thought to be due to an organic cause, psychological problems are often important contributing factors:

- the stress of performance pressure
- the stress of guilt about premarital sex, extramarital sex, or sex in general
- the stress of disease concerns, from the curable gonorrhea, to the incurable herpes, to the fatal AIDS
- the stress of abandonment fears, separation anxiety, or jealousy
- the stress of control struggles and manipulation tactics within relationships
- the stress of religious taboos
- the stress of pregnancy possibilities and birth control responsibilities
- the stress of intimacy and commitment issues
- the stress of the "madonna-whore" conflict; irreconcilable fantasies of "good girls who don't" and "bad girls who do"
- the stress of premature ejaculation or retarded ejaculation; problems hidden by erectile failure

Because erections are seen by most men as a demand for performance, no matter how impotence dysfunction starts out, it usually ends up as performance anxiety.

Treatment may have to address any or all of these psychody-

namics as well as refocus the man's attention on sensual pleasure and easy communication. Intercourse is proscribed (forbid-
den) until both erection and orgasm are no longer "goals" but,
rather, "bonuses" of pleasure play.

If you do not have immediate access to a sex therapist, schedule sensual sessions with your partner, but agree beforehand
that they won't include intercourse. This should help to eliminate performance pressure. Start by relaxing—showering
together, laughing together, talking together—and keep the
relaxed mood throughout. Take turns pleasuring each other so
that each of you will have a chance to focus fully on the sensations you are receiving. Don't worry about whether or not your
partner is having fun while you are being pleasured. Your partner will also have a turn and probably feels delighted at her
power to give you pleasure. Don't expect her to be a mind
reader; tell her what you enjoy. Don't confuse requests with
demands; requests are much more flattering. Do allow plenty of
time; after all, you're not trying to beat the clock. And do make
sure you are not tired; your aim is to feel sensual, not fall asleep.
Remember: You are not being called on to *do* anything, just to
have fun, and if an erection does happen to occur, all the better.

If your erections become more consistent after days or weeks
of this type of sensually focused intimacy, resume a full sex life
and know that occasional and mild erectile problems are common. If, however, the erectile problem persists or is also
accompanied by a loss of nocturnal erections, morning erections, or erections during masturbation, schedule a physical
checkup. When physical conditions such as diabetes, hormonal
deficiency, or drug-induced impotence (alcohol, high blood
pressure medication, certain tranquilizers) are ruled out or their
role defined, the next step is to consult with a sex therapist.
Sex therapists are usually psychiatrists, psychologists, social
workers, urologists, or gynecologists with special advanced
training in the techniques of sex therapy. They can help you
improve your sexual functioning if there is a physical basis or a
psychological one. Major medical centers, your physician, or
the American Association of Sex Educators, Counselors, and

Therapists in Washington, D.C., can provide the names of certified sex therapists to help you.

PREMATURE EJACULATION

Some cultures consider a quick orgasm more macho than others; this culture does not. Here, lasting long means being sexually strong. Lasting long means pleasuring your partner, and pleasuring yourself.

Some bodies respond orgasmically more quickly than others. This does not necessarily mean premature ejaculation is involved. Premature ejaculation is not measured in minutes; it is defined as ejaculation over which a man has *no sense of control*. This means that a man who *chooses* to come to orgasm quickly is not a premature ejaculator. A man who is *surprised* by his orgasm, even after many minutes of intercourse, could be. Having an orgasm "sneak up" on you may not only be the result of stress, but can certainly be the cause of stress as well.

Stress can accelerate premature ejaculation by distracting a man from his *premonitory sensations*. These are body signals that tell him that the first phase of his orgasm, the emission phase, is approaching. Once emission is completed and semen is deposited in the urethra, ejaculation is inevitable within a few seconds—and control is no longer likely.

To increase control, a man must pay particular attention to the sensation in his body as he becomes more and more aroused. If he recognizes those premonitory sensations that signal an approaching orgasm, he can slow his thrusting, alter the type of stimulation he is receiving, change position, or even pause until control is regained. If he is, instead, distracted by anxiety about premature ejaculation, or trying to distract himself in order to slow the premature ejaculation, the problem of loss of control is made worse. Each "failure" sets up more anticipatory stress for the next experience, and soon a man is likely to be so worried about satisfying his partner or embarrassing himself that his ability to focus and concentrate on what is going on in his body is lost.

The solution? Don't count backwards from one hundred or review baseball scores to reduce your arousal. Rather, *enjoy* your arousal. Pay more attention to it than ever before. Notice every sensation in your body so that your orgasm cannot catch you unaware. Practice by stimulating yourself until you begin to feel orgasmic sensations building. Stop movement immediately and wait until these sensations, but not your arousal, subside. Resume stimulation and repeat the stop-start pattern three times. Allow yourself to ejaculate on the third cycle. Then try this with four, five, even six cycles. You will begin to recognize your premonitory sensations more and more clearly. Then try the same stop-start pattern with your partner. You may be more distracted, self-conscious, or aroused trying this with a partner, so focus even more intently on your genital sensations, and make sure to provide her with her own "turn" to be pleasured to orgasm. A sex therapist can meet with you and your partner each week to talk about problems and progress.

RETARDED EJACULATION

Whereas premature ejaculation is probably the most common of the male sexual dysfunctions, retarded ejaculation is the least common. It means that while a man can have an erection and maintain it, he can't achieve an orgasm when he is with a partner. Most retarded ejaculators can masturbate to orgasm in private; some must just wait until the erection subsides on its own.

Retarded ejaculation may sound like a "good" dysfunction, turning a man into a super-stud capable of satisfying a woman endlessly. But sex therapy patients with this problem do not report feeling this way. Not being able to ejaculate is embarrassing, and waiting for an erection to subside is uncomfortable. For his partner, the stress may be even worse. She often feels that the man is holding back his orgasm, not aroused enough to come, or reluctant to put his pleasure in her care.

In contrast to premature ejaculation, in which stress can contribute to lack of control, in this case stress can contribute to the *overcontrol* that characterizes retarded ejaculation. The more life seems overwhelming, unpredictable, or demanding, the more any type of self-control may be expressed as a symbolic protest or statement of self-preservation. Ejaculatory control can become, for some men, that statement of self-control. Learning to allow spontaneous ejaculation to occur with a partner involves a series of "desensitization" steps. The orgasm must be disinhibited gradually—first in the presence of the partner, then by the partner herself, and finally by intercourse. Again, a certified sex therapist can help if you are experiencing this problem.

Male stress symptoms do not develop overnight. From this discussion it is clear that years of stress, many bouts of short-term stressors combined with long-term stressors, mix with a man's innate physical vulnerabilities, behaviors, and personal history to produce male stress symptoms. This process may begin as early as birth and continue in various forms throughout a man's life. There are some important early warning signals of stress and the damage it can inflict, however, and it's these that we'll look at in the next chapter.

4 EARLY WARNING SIGNALS: THEY CAN HELP SAVE YOUR LIFE

As I noted previously, the symptoms of stress more frequently suffered by women are painful, uncomfortable, and tend to compromise the quality of life. Those suffered by men, however, tend to kill. Important early signs of stress, which can contribute to or foreshadow these life-threatening symptoms, are very often ignored by men even though waiting might mean it's too late. Some of these early warning signs are physical symptoms, such as hyperventilation, chronic fatigue, heartburn, or nausea. Others are habitual behaviors, such as smoking, overeating, or drinking excessively. Still others are psychological dispositions, such as defiance, depression, or defensiveness. If you suffer from any one of these signs, it's time to intervene. You can't manage your stress once you are incapacitated. Pay attention to these early warning signs—they can help change the quality of your life, and they can help save your life.

PHYSICAL EARLY WARNING SIGNS

Before heart attacks there may be days of chest pains, months of cardiac arrhythmia (irregularities in rhythm), or even years of dizziness. Before ulcers there may be chronic heartburn or nausea. Before a stroke there may be gradually increasing blood pressure. Why are these important signals often ignored?

The men participating in the Male Stress Survey gave many answers. First, many respondents suggested that they may not be very sensitive to their own discomfort.

> "I don't do anything about pain until it gets so bad that I don't care anymore if I need an operation. Operations terrify me."

> "I feel like an old man when I pay attention to every ache and pain, so I ignore my pains. Maybe I should pay attention or I won't get to be an old man."

Research also supports the notion that men may have a higher pain threshold than women. This means that discomfort may have to build to higher levels before men become aware of it or check with their physicians.

Second, men admit that they are skilled at denial. More than 60 percent of the respondents said that when they are faced with physical problems that worry, frighten, or annoy them, they try to forget about them. Almost every one of these men volunteered a criticism of this dangerous approach, saying something like:

> "I'd be embarrassed if I was worried for nothing, so I don't even give a doctor a chance to laugh at me—as if he'd really laugh."

> "I know it's stupid, but I hate the thought of medicine and shots, so I want my physical problems to get better by themselves."

> "I'm not putting my body in a doctor's hands. So I guess it's not in anybody's hands."

Third, many men seem to set their physical health as a low priority.

"I know ignoring problems won't make them go away."
"I guess I'm not taking good enough care of myself."

Taking care of physical problems, in their minds, would leave less time to do the things they think *really* must be done. Taking care of their physical health would mean scheduling medical appointments when they see themselves as already overscheduled. Or attending to their body might mean a change in life-style, and "Who needs that?"

The answer, of course, is that *you* need that. You need regular checkups to monitor blood pressure changes, cardiac irregularities, and digestive problems; to assess the cause of headaches and backaches; to diagnose chronic fatigue, hyperventilation, muscle spasm, chest pains, dizziness, cold sweats, nausea, and increased allergic reactions.

You may also need to monitor signs of diseases and disorders that are not caused or aggravated by stress, but which can *create* stress by incapacitating physical movement, compromising sexual functioning, or diminishing intellectual concentration. Men, for example, can inherit hemophilia, some types of muscular dystrophy, and red-green color blindness, whereas women rarely do. Hemophilia is a blood-clotting disorder that affects approximately eight in ten thousand men. In Duchenne and Becker types of muscular dystrophy, muscle tissue does not maintain itself in males. And red-green color blindness, inconvenient but not health-threatening, is common to almost eight percent of all men and only one-tenth as many women.

Other disorders that are more frequently found in men than women include gout, hernias, and peptic ulcers. Ulcers have been described in Chapter 3 as a possible stress-caused disorder; gout and hernias can be described as stress-*causing* disorders. Gout refers to painful irritation of feet or hand joints by uric acid crystals. Excess uric acid, a by-product of the breakdown of protein for the body's use, can accumulate in crystal form in joints instead of being excreted in the urine. These crystals seem to form more readily in the presence of high alcohol intake, high-protein and organ-food diets, and lack of exercise. According to the authors of *Man's Body*, 95 percent of gout sufferers are men. Hernias, particularly those of the pelvic wall, are also men's problems. When the intestine pushes through the inguinal canal into the scrotum, the cause may be congenital, or due to weight gain or loss or the type of physical labor a man is more likely to do than a woman.

In addition to the physical conditions that signal stress or create stress, men must also recognize psychological and behavioral signs of stress.

BEHAVIORAL EARLY WARNING SIGNS

Because behavioral signs of stress are observable, repetitive, and usually consistent for each person, they are potentially the most useful of all early warning signals for the beginnings of the Male Stress Syndrome. Potentially useful, but too often unused! Compared to the Female Stress Syndrome findings, and to the women sampled about the Male Stress Syndrome, men sampled were far less aware of their own behavioral signs of stress. Most men noticed that they perspired more when stressed. Young men (eighteen to twenty-five) noticed that they were more irritable under stress. Men between twenty-five and forty years of age noticed that they were irritable and fidgety. Men in their next decade added that they had trouble falling asleep or staying asleep when they were stressed, and older men noticed sexual difficulties as yet another symptom. This relatively short list shows that there is a lamentable lack of self-awareness in this area among men.

On the other hand, the hundreds of women—wives, mothers, sisters, and friends—who participated in the Male Stress Survey noticed the following early warning signs of stress in their men:

1. Most frequently, women notice that men become *verbally abusive, curt,* or *critical* with their wives or children.

2. The second most frequently reported stress sign for men is *withdrawal.* Men seem to become more sullen, sulky, or silent; perhaps preoccupied.

3. Few men listed *overeating* as their own stress sign, but most women claim that the men in their lives often gain weight during periods of stress. When asked about overeating in direct interviews, men attributed their weight gains to lack of willpower, business lunches, boredom, or their wives' good cooking.

4. Similarly, women noticed that men *drink more alcohol* during stress periods. Men give other reasons for their drinking, but admit that their increased use does coincide with stress periods.

5. *Fatigue* is not among the most frequently noticed symptoms of male stress, but when it is mentioned, it usually heads the list. This would suggest that fatigue is not a universal symptom for all men, but that it is a consistent and important early warning sign for some men.

6. For other men, the reverse reaction to stress seems to be characteristic: *agitated activity.* These are men who seem to work off their tension. Throwing themselves into projects or work may distract them from their stress, channel the added adrenaline flowing, and provide an area of control and mastery in the midst of emotional chaos.

7. Among the quick fixes for stress, *smoking* is one of the most automatic. Smoking rates can easily double before men notice this stress sign. Many men told me that it took annoyed comments from co-workers bothered by their borrowing cigarettes, or that it took

their noticing that they had two cigarettes lit, to make them try to curb this behavior. The more stress they were under, however, the less successful they were in cutting back.

8. The most annoying male stress signals seemed to be *psychomotor habits:* foot-swinging, finger-tapping and knee-jiggling. Wives add that their husbands often keep them awake grinding their teeth at night. Husbands confirm that under stress they often have temporomandibular joint (jaw) pain in the mornings. Other wives say their husbands pace as if they are in a ten-foot race. Still other women complain that their fathers, sons, or husbands scratch itches that don't exist, smooth hairs that are already in place or have long since fallen out, or fix collars that are starched, buttoned down, and immobile.

9. *Somnambulistic withdrawal* sounds like a rare psychological disorder. Actually, it is a common stress reaction. It refers to the tendency to fall asleep when faced with stresses: marital arguments, plane flights, pre-income-tax preparations, or difficult decisions. Husbands say, "Who, me? Just tired." Wives say, "Yes, you. Now I know what to call it!"

10. Other men don't actually slip into sleep; they just become selectively deaf—they *tune out*. They hear but don't listen. In fact, they are dramatically distracted. They see but don't notice; they plan but don't remember.

11. Three times more males than females die in automobile accidents, and many of those accidents are a direct result of stress. *Reckless driving* may reflect anger, anxiety, impatience, impulsiveness, or depression, according to Ming T. Tsuang, professor of psychiatry at Harvard University. Driving after social stress, therefore, is five times more likely to lead to a fatal

accident. Many women report that they are terrified of being a passenger when their mate is stressed.

12. There is one sign of male stress which is consistently reported by mothers, daughters, wives, and lovers, and which is consistently omitted by males—yet they admit to it when confronted. It's *television tune-in*. Men don't always watch the program they tune in, but it pulls them out of social interaction and into distraction from stress.

13. *Facial gestures* associated with stress include: lip-chewing; tic-like spasms that pull lips into sneers, wrinkle noses, or raise eyelids until the whites are exposed; eye-blinking; lip-clicking; and repeated swallowing. The stressed male, however, seems to be the last to know what his face is doing!

14. The final behavioral sign that appeared frequently on the lists prepared by mothers, daughters, and mates was *increased spending*. Not uniquely male, of course, this early warning sign usually means the spender is feeling needy, wants a tangible symbol of his worth, or wants to receive "goodies" to counteract the "bad" in his life.

Rarely mentioned on the lists, but always mentioned in the research literature on stress, is the effect of stress on sexual behavior (as differentiated from sexual dysfunctions, which were discussed in Chapter 3). Sexual intimacy can reduce stress temporarily by providing pleasure; breaking into a work routine; mobilizing and utilizing adrenaline; offering a way to express adult affection, to be giving and to be appreciated; and affording an opportunity to relax. However, when stress relief becomes the motivation for sex, rather than the result of sex, another early warning signal is present.

Compulsive sex as the solution for many or all stresses is called satyriasis in men, and nymphomania in women. The problems that satyriasis creates outweigh the temporary stress relief it provides. Women complain that they feel their partners are making sexual demands, not sexual overtures; that they are merely convenient sexual objects rather than the object of sexual interest; and that they are likely to precipitate an anxiety attack if they say "no." Men who find that they masturbate or initiate sex compulsively under stress are equally upset by their own behavior since they have little sense of control. Now they must deal with the original stresses that triggered their sexual behavior, plus the stress that comes from feeling out of control.

A more common sign of stress, according to clinic reports, is a *loss of sexual interest.* A drop in the incidence of sexual fantasies, the frequency of lovemaking, the occurrence of morning erections or nocturnal erections, or an increase in the frequency of premature ejaculation or erectile problems may each be an early warning signal. Some couples realize this and look for the source of stress. Other couples do not, and focus on the sexual difficulty to the point where a sexual or marital problem is added to the stress mix.

THE DANGER OF STRESS DISTRACTIONS

Review the list of behavioral early warning signs of stress, and notice how many serve as *stress distractors.* Smoking, overeating, insomnia, increased spending, fights, sexual problems, and automobile accidents all set up their own stresses—sometimes more tangible and acceptable than the underlying stress sources. The overeater, for example, can worry about dieting and, at the same time, use those extra layers of fat to keep the world away, to provide an excuse for not being loved, or to explain achievement failures. Although overeating can start as an early warning stress symptom, it soon may become a stress distraction as well.

The use or abuse of psychotropic or "recreational" drugs functions very much the same way—as an early warning stress symptom that becomes so much of a problem that it distracts us from the original cause of the stress. Psychotropic drugs are drugs that alter behavior as a main effect. This definition would exclude aspirin and antibiotics, but would include:

1. *Sedative-hypnotics:* alcohol, barbiturates, and some tranquilizers. They induce drowsiness.

2. *Stimulants:* amphetamines, cocaine, nicotine, and caffeine. They increase alertness.

3. *Narcotics:* heroin, morphine, codeine, and the opiates. They produce euphoria.

4. *Hallucinogenics:* marijuana, hashish, mescaline, and LSD. They alter sensory input and reactions.

Any of the drugs in these four groups can be used as a temporary stress distraction. Getting the drugs can take time and effort. Taking the drugs can involve a ritual. Sharing the drugs may create a pseudo-subgroup that feels like a support network. Time on the drugs may be time away from the stress-causing problem. Time during withdrawal, psychological or physical, may be a time of preoccupation.

Although the psychotropic effect of each group of drugs is different, the use of any of them is usually *stress-induced* and definitely *stress-generating.* The sedative-hypnotics, for example, are attractive to men feeling anxious or hyperactive because of stress, but they produce drunkenness, hangover, convulsions, coma, and even death at increased dosages. The stimulants are attractive to men struggling with depression, but they overwork the fight and flight system even more quickly and more fatally than does long-term stress. Narcotics may dull the psychological pain of stress, but they are quickly physically addicting. The hallucinogenics provide not only a psychedelic ("mind-bending") trip away from real-life stress, but they also produce psychotomimetic ("psychosis-imitating") experiences that can be stressful enough to induce suicide.

None of the behaviors that signal the onset of stress can be ignored. They are not behaviors that address the source of stress or serve to diminish it or its effects. In fact, these early warning signals usually create their own stress consequences, compounding the original problem. Drug addiction, sexual disinterest, and family conflict may preoccupy a stressed man enough to distract him from his stress, but not constructively. The physical effects of long-term stress on the male body are devastating, as I've described. Behavioral early warning signals must be recognized or they, too, will affect the male body. The psychological effects of long-term stress on the male sense of self can be equally devastating.

PSYCHOLOGICAL EARLY WARNING SIGNS

The psychological signs of stress that men most frequently exhibit may precede their awareness of stress. I call these psychological signs the "six D's": defensiveness, depression, disorganization, defiance, dependency, and decision-making difficulties. Any one of these early warning signs may first appear in mild form or intermittently. As stress continues, so will the psychological signal, and its severity will probably increase.

Some men will show one particular psychological stress sign, others will experience two, three, or all of these early warning signals.

It was almost noon and Evan had not yet decided how he wanted to use the day. He knew he should prepare his taxes, could play handball, might have enough time to run up to a wrecking company warehouse for a mantelpiece, or would be able to catch the last quarter of the game he had bet on. He wondered at his own indecision. It felt unfamiliar in general, but increasingly noticeable during the last few weeks. Maybe it's because Susan is away more now, he mused. Couldn't be, he concluded, and sat down to read the newspaper, again.

Manny had the keys to his car in his hand one minute ago, and now they were gone. He had not left the room, yet they seemed to have disappeared from the face of the earth. His absentmindedness made him angry. He snapped at his mother, who was passing through the room, and then indignantly denied that he was irritable when she confronted him. He wished briefly that he was still just a college student, but covered up that wish with a display of paper-sorting and briefcase-packing. He still didn't know what he wanted to say at the meeting that morning, and didn't even care, but he knew he had better find his keys soon!

Evan was showing one early warning stress signal, decision-making difficulties; Manny was showing many—defensiveness, disorganization, defiance, dependency, depression, and decision-making difficulties. Check the chart below for the stress signs you have experienced or observed. Any of these psychological signs indicates the beginnings of the Male Stress Syndrome. More than one indicates *moderate to high stress*.

_____ *Defensiveness*

Defensiveness reflects the unrealistic expectation that a man must "be a man." That is, he should not show weakness; he should not be touched by stress. Sometimes this defensiveness is a public display rehearsed for years. Sometimes it is also a private conviction and leads to destructive self-blame and overly critical self-evaluation.

_____ *Depression*

Underlying the feeling of depression is usually anger or loss. Under stress, men feel angry that they could not control all the aspects of their lives, and they feel a loss of their sense of control. The physical and behavioral symptoms, furthermore, may overwhelm them. If professional help is needed (medical or psychiatric), their depression may initially deepen.

_____ *Disorganization*   Stress preoccupies and diminishes concentration. The resulting disorganization can show up as sloppiness, absentmindedness, or lapses in judgment.

_____ *Defiance*   Some men fight back when they feel stressed, even if there is no actual focus for their defiance. They may challenge "authority" figures, become argumentative, or deliberately dissent arbitrarily.

_____ *Dependency*   Many men regress under stress. They would love to be saved and to be taken care of, but rarely admit this fantasy to others—perhaps not even to themselves. Often they add to their stress by denying or feeling guilty about this need.

_____ *Decision-Making Difficulties*   Feeling stressed usually means feeling a lack of control, choice, or preparation in a situation. Making decisions, even minor decisions, under such conditions becomes very difficult.

If you and your mate filled out the checklist, compare your results. A spouse can often provide very valuable feedback. Perhaps you thought that no one in the world knows when you are suffering, anxious, or stressed. Perhaps you thought no one would care if you were. Now is the time to discuss this concern with those close to you so that at least the added stress of feeling isolated will be alleviated. Your mate, your mother, your father, your friends, and I give you permission to feel dependent, depressed, disorganized, defensive, defiant, or undecided while you are under high stress. Now you must give *yourself* permission.

Of course, permission to feel psychologically distressed is not the same thing as permission to act out your distress. Working through and working out stress involves problem-solving, self-awareness, realistic action, exercise, and even relaxation techniques. *Acting out* stress, as Manny did, refers to behavior that provides only momentary catharsis (release)—often at your own or someone else's expense. For example:

> Thirty-three-year-old Scott was on his way to an appointment with a new plant manager when his car got a flat tire. Not only was he going to be late, but he was going to be dirty. Cursing, he eased the car onto the shoulder of the road, got out, slammed the door shut, and started the tire-changing routine. He was, of course, late for the appointment, and unfortunately, he did not get the position he wanted. He arrived home wanting to let off steam, yell, find someone to blame. He looked for an excuse to shout until he found one. He convinced himself that his wife was starting up with him until he thought about it later. He had not solved the original problem, but had instead created a new one. His wife was now angry and defensive, and he felt alone with his misery and guilt.

Actually, the case of Scott is not unlike the old story of the man who is yelled at by his boss, so yells at his wife when he gets home, who yells at their son, who yells at the dog, who chases the cat . . . The problem with acting out frustration in this way is that research clearly demonstrates that aggressive behavior serves mainly as a rehearsal for more aggressive behavior. Furthermore, you have now provided a model for your spouse and children. The more you let your stress out on others, the more practiced you will be at it and the more likely they are to do the same. Watch for the following indications of "acting out" in yourself and others:

- inappropriate or exaggerated anger
- deliberate lack of cooperation, or "nay-saying"
- uncharacteristic fault-finding
- impossible demands
- unprovoked sarcasm

These patterns indicate attitudes that may be early warning

stress signals if they are uncharacteristic and recent. If, on the other hand, these patterns are characteristic and long-standing, your stress is probably chronic. If your life circumstances are the problem, make some choices and changes. If choices and changes are not a realistic alternative, read Chapter 9 on living with stress. If neither your perspective nor your behavior changes, you should consider professional counseling, since you are clearly generating as many problems as you are reacting to.

EARLY WARNING STRESS CHECKLIST

Take the following test from the Male Stress Survey, which over five hundred men have already taken, and then compare your results to theirs. Check all items that are true for you:

_____ When I am under stress I eat more.

_____ When I am under stress I eat much less.

_____ When I am under stress I smoke more.

_____ When I am under stress I drink more alcohol.

_____ When I am under stress I have trouble falling asleep.

_____ When I am under stress I have trouble staying asleep.

_____ When I am under stress I become more irritable and impatient.

_____ When I am under stress I have less of a sense of humor.

_____ When I am under stress I have less interest in sex.

_____ When I am under stress I become disorganized or forgetful.

_____ When I am under stress I become quiet and withdrawn.

_____ When I am under stress I become pessimistic or depressed.

_____ When I am under stress I behave compulsively or repetitively.

_____ When I am under stress I become critical of others.

_____ When I am under stress I become restless and fidgety.

_____ When I am under stress I work myself harder.

_____ When I am under stress I grind my teeth or clench my jaw.

This checklist was designed to reflect the behavioral and psychological stress symptoms that have been reviewed in this chapter. To round out the picture, take another look at the lists of physical symptoms on pages 30–31, and note again your responses to them. Because this test is an instrument for self-assessment, scores are meaningless—each and every symptom deserves your full attention. However, the most frequently checked behavioral items on the Male Stress Survey, combining men's and women's responses, turned out to be the statements suggesting that men under stress:

- become irritable and impatient
- become withdrawn
- increase their eating
- increase their smoking
- increase their drinking
- show activity changes: fatigue or hyperactivity
- develop sleeping problems
- become restless and fidgety

Is this your pattern, too? In addition, when men were given a chance to write in stress symptoms not mentioned on the checklist, further early warning signs appeared. Men said that under stress they:

- become more self-critical
- ignore their friends
- feel more jealous and suspicious
- tend to stutter or trip over their words
- repeat themselves
- develop temporary sexual dysfunctions

The physical stress signals most frequently checked by men were:

- headaches
- nausea
- heartburn
- muscle aches, particularly backaches
- high blood pressure

When asked to write in physical stress signs not mentioned on the checklist, they added:

- dry mouth, scratchy eyes
- muscle stiffness and clumsiness
- shivering or shaking
- increased perspiration
- erratic breathing

Taking the time to think about your own early warning stress signals will, I hope, give you more time to reduce and manage your stress before you are incapacitated or your functioning is permanently altered. Remember, increased *control, choice,* and *predictability* decrease stress. This applies to stress symptoms as well. The sooner you can recognize your early warning signs, the more you can control your stress levels, choose alternatives to stressful situations, and anticipate what will happen next if you don't!

PERSONAL PATTERNS

The question I was asked most frequently by the men who were surveyed for this study was "Why me?" They were asking why they developed headaches but not backaches, or high blood pressure but not ulcers. How are individual differences between stress symptom patterns explained? Why are some symptoms so common and others so unique or idiosyncratic?

Personal patterns of early warning signals seem to be the product of many interacting factors. The most primary will always be the particular *vulnerabilities* of each body. For example, men in general seem to have a cardiovascular system that is vulnerable to stress; but any man in particular may be more or less vulnerable than the average in that area. Thus there are men who may never develop heart disease despite enormous stress, and others who will have their first heart attack by age forty. Similarly, few men develop true anorexia under stress, but any given individual male may be predisposed to this eating disturbance. Under pressure, then, weak links break first. And early warning stress signals are often information about our body's weak links.

Personal stress symptom patterns are also the product of the *strengths* of each body, as well as its weaknesses. The more that a particular body system or organ can withstand stress effects, the more likely that another system or organ will eventually show a sign of stress instead. In such cases, the symptoms will appear later rather than earlier, since the site was not particularly vulnerable. In such cases the symptom will probably be less rather than more severe, since the site was not particularly vulnerable. And in such cases the symptom will appear only after more, rather than less, stress, since the site was not particularly vulnerable.

Personal stress experiences also seem to contribute to personal stress symptom patterns, individualizing each incidence of the Male Stress Syndrome. Although Hans Selye originally described the autonomic fight and flight reaction as nonspecific, current research suggests that each type of stressor produces *subtle but specific* autonomic differences. Anger or fight situations, for example, seem to stimulate the release of norepinephrine, while fear or flight situations stimulate the release of epinephrine. Similarly, anger seems to produce increased blood pressure, whereas fear seems to produce increased respiration and perspiration. Individual life histories and stressor sensitivities, then, may also be influencing the personal pattern of stress signals that emerges.

Here are some other factors that probably promote particular early warning signals in particular men:

1. His *age* at the time or times of stress. At fifteen stress may produce a headache; at fifty it may produce a heart attack.

2. The state of his body's *health* at the time of stress. If a particular organ or system is weakened by a disease or virus, it will of course be more vulnerable to stress.

3. His *personality* may predispose him to particular symptoms. Psychoanalytic theory suggests that asthma is an expression of repressed crying, compulsive behavior is an attempt to block angry action, and overeating is a type of self-feeding that indicates dependency needs. Many case studies support this hypothesis, but few correlational studies statistically agree.

4. A man's *learning history* can significantly influence his stress responses, both physical and behavioral. Some experts suggest, for example, that if stomachaches earned him more attention than sprained ankles in his early years, he may be more apt to be an ulcer victim in later years than an accident victim. If shouting was more frequently reinforced by attention than sulking when he was a boy, verbal abusiveness may be more his stress style than withdrawal as a man.

5. Male *role models* teach stress reaction by example. Children imitate behavior reinforced by others. As we know, children rarely do as we *say*—they unfortunately usually do as we *do!* Boys who were abused by stressed fathers are very likely to become child abusers themselves as adults. On the other hand, children who hear their fathers verbalize their anxieties and see them take steps toward reducing their stress have been taught a valuable first lesson in stress survival.

6. Some *individual differences* in stress symptom development are not easily explained but are very obvious.

It is obvious that each male seems to have his own threshold for psychosomatic reactions and his own combination of stress variables that can push him toward that threshold. In other words, for each man:

- The duration of the stress needed to activate a warning symptom can vary.

- The frequency of stress experiences that can be tolerated can vary.

- The intensity of the stress as it is subjectively experienced is different for each man and can influence the appearance of a stress symptom.

- The confluence or sequence of stresses can lead to different stress outcomes. If the death of a parent precedes a minor accident, the victim may feel far more anxious and dependent than he would, had the preceding stress been assuming a larger mortgage!

- The symbolic meaning of a particular stress to a particular person can affect its stress impact.

Early warning signals, then, not only help men to head off the more serious consequences of the Male Stress Syndrome, they also can help men learn about their own emotional learning history, their own readiness to cope or capitulate to particular stresses, their own symptom patterns, their own psychological and physical vulnerabilities, and their own personality profiles. Studying them can teach men which symptoms they learned and which they inherited. The former they can moderate; the latter they must monitor.

5 GROWING UP MALE

MANY STAGES OF A WOMAN'S LIFE ARE MORE SHARPLY DEMARKED BY changes in her body than are similar stages of a man's life. Menstruation leaves a woman with no doubt that her puberty has begun; pregnancy signals the beginning of her parenthood; and menopause surely reminds her that she has reached midlife and that her reproductive stage is over. Changes in a man's life are usually more biologically gradual and psychologically subtle. As puberty begins, the boy starts to develop a deeper voice, more body hair, and viable sperm, but these develop slowly and there is no one dramatic moment to mark the "onset" of puberty. He does not awaken one morning to a new beard or new voice. His body does not tell him, usually, when he is ready to become a father or if he no longer has enough sperm to become a father. His sexual functioning may change as he grows older, but this usually doesn't happen suddenly or predictably, and sometimes there is hardly any change at all.

Since a man cannot always rely on his body to tell him what stage of life he has entered or is leaving, or predict what will happen to him next, he must find an alternative to the biological clock. He usually sets an *achievement clock* going instead.

Jeff is twenty-three years old and has just finished an MBA degree. How does he see his future? "By thirty I want to be married and in a career that is taking off. By forty, I should have some children, maybe own a house, and at least have a 'title' at work. By fifty, I think I should have it all: some luxuries; some long vacations; some power. Beyond fifty? Until then, and maybe even then, I don't want to look ahead." After fifty, he says, he fears decline. After sixty, he fears disability. After seventy, he fears death.

When men don't achieve as they expect to, they feel stress. When men become too ill or too old to perform occupationally, sexually, or athletically, they feel stress. When men cannot or do not control their outer life circumstances, they feel stress. This is a double stress jeopardy: Men must deal not only with the realities of life events and life changes, but they must also deal with the special meanings that these events and changes have for them. They may feel that bad luck is failure, that unpredictability is the result of a lack of foresight, and that others' choices are the result of their own lack of control.

Where do these notions of achievement come from? Why do Jeff and other men particularly fear becoming ill or too old to perform? When do men learn that controlling their outer life can make them less anxious about their inner life? The starting place for all of this seems to be in the home, and in the way boys are raised from the moment of their birth.

A BOY IS BORN

The average American male is born weighing 7½ pounds, a half pound heavier than the average newborn female. His heart and lungs are larger and he's usually born earlier. He has more testosterone pumping through his bloodstream. He "startles" more readily than female neonates, and makes more movements per minute. Although he is probably larger and more active at birth, he is at higher risk of death by miscarriage or death by birth. Though the fact that he is biologically vulnerable is bad news, the good news is that he is almost certain to be *wanted* by his parents. Female infanticide is an historical fact, but male infanticide is almost unheard of in any country. Males are valued for their ability to carry on the family name, defend the family honor, increase the family's economic base, or inherit and run the family enterprise.

The average American male grows from 7½ pounds at birth to weigh about 165 pounds as an adult. In between, he not only shows characteristic physical changes, but seems to exhibit some characteristically male behavioral changes as well. This doesn't mean that an individual boy might not show unique patterns of development, or might not be calmer or quieter than many. This doesn't mean that males and females necessarily start out differently or need end up differently. What it means is that whether or not genetic sex-linked differences influence emotions, cognition, or capacity, four other factors definitely do: parental expectations, modeling, sensitization, and media messages.

PARENTAL EXPECTATIONS

The capacities that develop most fully in people are those that are reinforced first at home. The ways in which parents treat boys influence the ways in which boys treat themselves. Early messages become internalized messages, familiar messages— they become part of the boy's introduction to the world and to his concept of self.

Among the traditional expectations parents have for their sons are:

- Boys are expected to be stronger than girls.
- Boys are expected to be less emotional and intuitive.
- Boys are expected to be more aggressive and impulsive.
- Boys are expected to be active and alert.
- Boys are expected to be more self-reliant than girls.
- Boys are expected to take everything apart.

- Boys are expected to stay awake longer and nap less.
- Boys are expected to play war, not house.

According to studies by developmental psychologist Michael Lewis and many others, these expectations are reflected in the way parents handle their sons:

- Fathers will play roughhouse games with their infant sons more readily than with their infant daughters.

- Both mothers and fathers will respond less to their infant sons' vocalizations than to their daughters' sounds. They both respond more to his attempts to grasp, crawl, and walk.

- Parents let boys roam farther than girls in playgrounds and yards.

- Parents push boys into activities that frighten them more readily than they push girls.

It may, of course, be true that males have a higher activity level than females in general, and that females respond more readily to voices than males in general. But these tendencies become specifically directed into sex-role behaviors by both fathers and mothers. This socialization starts at birth because the parents' expectations for a boy's behavior were established even before he was born.

MODELING

"When I grow up I want to be like Daddy." It's a natural feeling and usually starts no later than the middle of the second year. Even nine-month-old babies can distinguish males from females, and by two years of age the child has a good sense of his own gender identity.

According to psychologist Jerome Kagan, in his book *Personality Development*, the little boy is busy identifying with, or "modeling" himself after, his father for four reasons:

- He has noticed that they are physically the same, and that his Mommy and sister are different.

- He can identify with his father's emotions since he has already been encouraged to express and repress the same ones.

- He wants to be able to do what his father can do; and to be rewarded, therefore, as his father is rewarded.

- He feels comfortable imitating his father's mannerisms since they are familiar to him and draw his father and mother closer to him.

Once a boy has managed some modeling, the results are remarkably stable. In fact, psychophysiologists Anka Ehrhardt and John Money find that by two years of age, reassigning sexual gender identity is unsuccessful or severely stressful. That is, when children who are really genetically female were raised as boys because of genital abnormalities, they are better adjusted when they are allowed to continue their lives as males than when they are told that they must now start to think of themselves as female. Ehrhardt and Money's fascinating book, *Man and Woman, Boy and Girl*, explores the current research into the interaction of biological factors and modeling.

A baby boy is not only being treated differently than a baby girl, then; he is identifying with a different model. He will learn how to be a male by seeing what other males do—particularly his father. So, if Daddy handles frustration with aggression, his son will try that too. If Daddy expresses disapproval by withdrawing, his son will try that too. If Daddy holds in his sadness, his son may think he should do the same.

Yet if Daddy is rewarding and nurturing, his son is likely to develop more "masculine" behaviors than the sons of fathers who are less warm! Researchers E. M. Hetherington, D. Lynn, and L. F. Distler, each in separate studies, found the same results: the more the father shows love and praise as well as punishment, the more of an influence he will have on his son. This is vital information for every father. Hugging, sharing, and sympathizing with your son will encourage his male modeling more than will direct efforts at sex-typed behavior. In fact, a nurturing father seems to produce both a more masculine son and a more feminine daughter!

SENSITIZATION

The child who touches a hot stove once is likely to stay away from stoves for a long time. He has been "sensitized" to them. Similarly, boys and girls can be sensitized to social situations that produce intense short-term stress or upsetting long-term stress.

Joshua, three years old, scraped his knee while playing with two five-year-old boys. He saw the blood, felt the pain, and started to cry. His playmates started chanting, "Baby, baby, baby!" Older boys hanging around started to laugh. His aunt hit him for making so much noise and told him that big boys don't carry on like that. Joshua stopped crying but did not go back into the game. When he got home that afternoon, he kicked his puppy as hard as he could.

Joshua had become sensitized to shame. He didn't have to be *told* anything; he learned his shame lesson from mocking glances and group rejection. His anger at the tyrants who would not let him express his hurt feelings distracted him from his shame. But that means that Joshua would now be sensitized to feeling the anger of frustration, too. Both feelings, shame and anger, would be forever familiar. He will probably try to avoid both. Both will remind him of how it feels to be three years old: powerless, and pained.

Many boys become sensitized to rejection by trying to give or receive affection and being met with rigid, awkward responses from their fathers. Their fathers' embarrassment makes the boys feel embarrassed as well—embarrassed by their own behavior. They will try to control that behavior next time, and the relief they will feel when they do will further reinforce emotional constriction. The lesson sinks in quickly and the sensitization to embarrassment may last a lifetime.

"Mommy's little boy" or "Daddy's big man": either script is too rigid and stereotyped to fit reality. Sons may meet either or both role requirements, but free-floating hostility will be the price. Current research suggests that boys are now being raised in a climate that permits greater emotional expression than ever before. If this is true, it is likely to produce men who are more sensitive and less "sensitized," and it's likely that the fathers of this generation are working hard to overcome their own sensitization. The men of tomorrow may suffer less from the Male Stress Syndrome.

MEDIA MESSAGES

Turn on a prime-time television program, drop in to see a blockbuster film, scan a bestselling spy novel, or check out the latest video games. What's the message for men? Fast-thinking, fast-driving, and fast-hitting men win. What do they win? The wallet, the woman, and the war. And how much of this do children absorb? All of it. In fact, Jean Piaget, the pioneer of the study of children's cognitive development, found that children do not fully understand the nature of dreams, fantasies, and fictions until they are about nine or ten years old. By then, the average child will have seen the destruction of more than 6,000 people on TV; by the time he is fifteen years old, he will have seen 13,000 or more violent TV deaths.

Twenty-one years ago, the Surgeon General linked television to aggressive behavior. Thousands of studies have confirmed the link between media input and children's violent behavior.

- In the 1960s, social psychologists Albert Bandura, D. Ross, and A. Ross found that 79 percent of children who watched a cartoon with aggression and violence imitated some of the behavior while playing afterward. This finding seemed to be borne out in the case of a five-year-old who set a house afire, and killed his toddler sibling in the process, after he viewed the MTV cartoon series *Beavis and Butthead*, on which a character frequently plays with matches.

- Social learning expert R. M. Liebert reported years ago that children remember the acts of aggression in stories more vividly than they remember whether the "bad guys" were punished or not.

- A report issued in 1993 by the American Psychological Association's Commission on Violence said that viewing violence increases violence and leads to emotional desensitization toward violence.

- A twenty-two-year study of 875 children first observed at age eight showed that boys who were not unusually aggressive at school but who watched great amounts of violent TV programs, grew up to be as violence-prone as the eight-year-olds who were the most aggressive school bullies.

- Television is not the only culprit, and young boys are not the only victims. In 1993, for example, there was a small rash of "copycat" incidents in which teenage boys were either injured or killed while lying in the center of busy roads in imitation of a scene from a movie about college football called *The Program*.

The media tell children about more than violence. They also teach us that men are supposed to be competitive high achievers who keep their emotions in check in order to get the job done. In 1979, sociologist L. Weitzman and his associates studied children's books for preschoolers and found that the characters were usually highly sex-typed. And even though newer studies of children's books show some improvement, general stereotypes remain: competitive, active boys; dependent, passive girls. So in books Dick still goes to the office with Daddy instead of baking cookies with Mommy or going to the office with her. Novels for teenagers still tell of the underdog learning to fight back to win the football game or prettiest girl on campus. In films, men still are portrayed as hunters, fighters, natural athletes, avengers, scientists, leaders, and supernatural heroes. In fact, my daughter, when she was young, told me that she was going to be a nurse and her boy cousin would be a doctor when they grew up, because only men are doctors—despite the fact that her mother, grandmother, and godmother all carry the title of doctor and work in hospitals!

Even advertisements reinforce the notion that men must be

high performers. They compete hard, and then they can drink beer. They work hard and then eat gourmet. They play hard and then dress well. On film this behavior can be fun to watch; on television it can sell commercial time; in books, it can involve us in a fantasy. In real life, however, such unrealistic notions of achievement can create stress, even kill.

The legacy of the boy's early training through modeling, sensitization, and media messages is the man's stress. If the boy is taught to dread failure, the man suffers from performance anxiety. He wants to achieve and win satisfaction and praise, but fears the shame and guilt of falling short of his goal. If the boy is taught to compete to win, the man suffers from competitive compulsions. He can't stop comparing himself to others and protecting himself from others long enough to *relax* with others. If the boy is taught to repress feelings that are "unmanly," the man suffers from emotional channeling. He guides all his emotional energy into those few outlets that are acceptable.

> Ray rushed through the kitchen on his way to the garage, but slowed down to give his ten-year-old son a gentle slap on the back. "Do well today," he said; then left. Gene was on time as Ray drove by his first carpool stop, and looking well despite his recent surgery. As Gene settled into the passenger side of the front seat, Ray leaned over and gave him a warm slap on the back. "Nothing can keep you down," Ray said. Gene smiled. Ray thanked the parking attendant in the lot for saving a front space with a hearty backslap, and then entered his office building. "Where's the mail?" he asked Joey ten minutes later. "I forgot yours," Joey sheepishly mumbled. Ray sent him out the door for the mail with a slap on the back.

For Ray, a backslap is an acceptable emotional channel. But how narrow a channel it is. A hug or handshake might often be a more accurate expression of his feelings. Or have his feelings themselves become restricted to those that can be channeled into a backslap?

Performance anxiety, competitive compulsions, and emotional channeling create demands that men try to meet. Meeting these demands creates stress, and we see that the Male Stress Syndrome can begin very early indeed.

TODDLER TO TEENS

Although nobody really knows what goes on in an infant's mind, we can assume that stress starts when life begins. T. Berry Brazelton of Boston's Children's Hospital, for example, speculates that infant stress can come from boredom, meaning lack of stimulation, or frustration, meaning lack of skill mastery. The infant's early warning symptom? Rhythmic rocking back and forth, or repeated rolling of the head.

EARLY STRESSES

As the infant boy grows older, the causes of stress and the signs of stress become more easily identified. David McClelland and David Pilon of Harvard University suggest, for example, that the stress of very strict toilet training and feeding schedules produces children who are used to living up to a lot—and, later, adults who have a driven need for achievement. On the other hand, they find that very lax parenting when it comes to aggression produces boys who are used to doing things *their* way and who must be in control as adults. Either way, the message is the same: Assert yourself.

And how early does emotional channeling begin? A psychologist videotaped forty-eight male and female two- and three-year-olds while they took care of dolls and as their parents looked on. The parents praised the girls, saying such things as, "You're such a good mommy," but did not encourage such nurturing in the boys. Andy's story is extreme, but it makes the point.

"When I was five years old I fell down some stairs. I wasn't hurt at all, just a little bruised. But I guess I was scared and shaken. I started to cry. Just then my father came home and found out what had happened. He said only girls cried. So for all the next week he made me wear girls' dresses. And he made sure that I was outside the house a lot, where people could see me. I'm thirty now. After three years of psychotherapy, I can finally cry again."

Most parents do not go this far; but many fathers will do their best to insist that their sons be "all man." Wallace was only seven when this happened:

"I was an only child and a late child. I think my father didn't really know what to do with me. We were at the beach, and he put me on his shoulders and began to walk into the water. I don't know why, but I became terrified. Maybe I thought he was taking me away from my mother—or from the whole world. I started screaming, but he kept walking further in, as if he didn't hear me. I was pulling his hair and screaming and pleading. It didn't make any difference. Finally, when he couldn't go any deeper himself, he came back to shore. I was freezing and shivering and scared out of my wits. He looked at me and said that he'd take me and throw me into the water if I ever did that again."

When the toddler leaves the house, he enters school; the expectations of his teachers now converge with those of his parents and reinforce each other. Again the boy is encouraged in his competitive compulsions, his performance anxiety, and his emotional channeling.

Boys are the favored gender, at home and at school. Social scientists Myra and David Sadker, who have researched gender bias in classrooms throughout the U.S., point out that boys are more likely than girls to rise to the top of the class *and* to fall to the bottom. That's because boys dominate girls in the classroom and consequently get more teacher attention. When boys cross the line of acceptable behavior by raising their hands, shouting out the answers, and sometimes even interrupting the teacher in midsentence they are remembered for all the wrong reasons. In fact, so pervasive is the concern over male misbehavior that even when a boy and a girl are involved in an identical infraction of the rules, the male is more likely to get the penalty.

All in all, academic stress seems greater for boys: from elementary school through high school, boys receive lower report card grades; are more likely than girls to be grade repeaters and dropouts; are nine times more likely to suffer from hyperactivity; and comprise 71 percent of all school suspensions.

At school, with friends, and at home, the message still seems often to be that boys are supposed to remain within gender lines and avoid, above all, acting like a "girl."

PEER PRESSURE

The lessons of assertion, achievement, and nonweakness, learned from parents, teachers, and other adult media models, are reinforced by peers. It's not only the coach who emphasizes winning, it's the other boys as well—and they can be more demanding, critical, and cruel than any adult.

A preteen boy today spends approximately twice as much time with his "best friend" and groups of friends as he does with his parents. In a study of over seven hundred sixth-graders, J. Condry, Jr., and associates found that most of the children spent only two or three hours a day with their parents over the weekend! Is this stressful for the boy? Not necessarily, since friends are an important source of self-esteem, feedback, and validation. But peers can present values that are in conflict with parental teachings, and *boys are more influenced by their friends than are girls* (M. Siman). As Papalia and Olds put it:

> From time immemorial, parents have worried about the friends their children are seeing, with some justification....It is usually in the company of friends that children engage in petty shoplifting, smoke their first cigarettes, chug-a-lug their first cans of beer, sneak into the movies, and do other antisocial acts.

Unfortunately, it is the boys who are the least secure, the most stressed, the most dependent, and who are the most vulnerable to peer pressure and peer displeasure. They are the ones who can least tolerate being shut out, unpopular, or criticized. If they become defensive, they are sure to be picked on. If they become withdrawn, they are sure to be isolated. If they become aggressive, they are sure to be ganged up on. If they become anxious, they are sure to be teased. So they often conform instead—they are angry, perhaps, but they conform. And once again, free-floating hostility may combine with emotional channeling, performance pressure, and control compulsions to produce early male stress.

The boy growing from toddler to teen has to deal with two inner stresses as well as the stresses associated with school and peers. To function well as a teen and then as an adult, he must begin the tasks of separation from his parents and control of his aggression.

SEPARATION ANXIETIES AND PROBLEMS

All children must periodically separate from their parents. They build their own skills and want to test them. It starts with the infant learning to toddle away from Mommy, and proceeds to the high-school or college graduate leaving home for his or her own apartment.

This separation, though healthy, is always somewhat frightening. Therefore, it usually follows a leave/return pattern. The toddler walks away from his mother, but soon comes back to see if she is still there—just in case! The nursery school child looks forward to playing with his friends, but also to coming home. So the boy detaches himself to explore the world, and reattaches himself for a greater security.

Unfortunately, some boys may be discouraged by their mothers, or their fathers, in the reattachment process. For example, they may have been taught that they are not *supposed* to feel frightened or insecure. In other families, emotional attachment may not have been encouraged in the first place, so the boy does not feel secure enough to explore. He will still be waiting to get what he needs at home while other children have moved on to sports, academics, and friendships. Still other boys may not be sure that their parents will be there when they return— figuratively or literally. Fear of parental divorce or parental separation can certainly interfere with the child's ability to separate. Finally, some mothers may unknowingly signal their sons to stay too close. These are boys whose fathers may be absent, or who may be taught that their fathers are inadequate and that they themselves must act as a substitute—an overwhelming idea for a child!

> Ken and Ron are brothers, but their age difference is as great as their family experience. Ken grew up in the late 1950s. His father earned enough for the whole family, and his mother enjoyed being a full-time, first-time mother. His father was energetic and loving and, unknowingly, fatally ill. He died in 1964, one year after Ron was born.
>
> The boys' mother grieved for years. She became anxious that something would happen to her baby whenever she left the house. As he grew, she feared that he would be hurt whenever *he* left the house. She often repeated to friends and family that she was not left well-provided-for, and worried about the boys' welfare if she should die also. Ken responded by getting a job while he was in college and contributing to the household support. Ron responded by developing colitis attacks every time he wanted to leave the house to play. Soon the attacks began to prevent him from leaving for school as well. Although his mother was upset about his pain, she was relieved to have him close and in her care. She liked to be needed, and Ron certainly felt that he needed her.

How does the young man who has separation problems handle this early stress? He cannot turn to his parents, and he has probably not been able to bond with friends; so he turns to control, again. If he can't go back to his mother or father, he must either never leave emotionally, or he must set up his life so he can feel in total control wherever he is. Any change will be stressful, therefore, because it threatens the order he has imposed on his life.

CHANNELING OF AGGRESSION

Another focus of control for the young boy is control of his aggressive impulses. At the same time that he is learning that he must control aggression in general, he is learning that specific forms of aggression are acceptable. Hitting may be disallowed and shouting frowned upon, but sports are fine, and so is practically any kind of academic or skills competition. Thus aggression is channeled into competition, and competition is channeled into achievement.

Problems arise, however, when parents and teachers can't or won't set limits. Some parents and teachers get a vicarious kick out of a child's aggression. It is as if their own squelched impulses are finally being projected into the open. Alternately, parents and teachers might be overly frightened of their own aggression and, therefore, of the child's.

> Dinner was a silent time for Greg. His father would pronounce his opinions during the meal as if he were delivering a sermon. Greg would want to discuss things, disagree with or question his father, but he learned that even the slightest hint of dialogue would be considered disrespect. His father never raised his voice when he was displeased with Greg. He would clench his teeth, breathe deeply, close his eyes, then slowly pronounce a punishment. Sometimes Greg would try to imagine what his father's rage would be like if it were really let loose. Too terrible, he decided, to risk. He wondered silently what his own would be like. Too terrible, he knew.

Overcontrol sends the message that angry impulses are terrifying rather than manageable. Soon the child is repressing, not rechanneling, his aggression. With no outlet, hostility can only build and contribute to the Male Stress Syndrome to come.

"RIGHTS" OF PASSAGE

Parents can help their sons pass through these potentially difficult learning stages by being armed with information that will permit them to manage stress in later life as well as now. Parents can also help themselves deal with the Male Stress Syndrome by recognizing which of these early stresses still sensitize and affect their functioning now. You and your son must both move on.

- Let him cry and be frightened when it is appropriate. If you give him permission to have these feelings, he can give *himself* permission. There will be times when this will help preserve his health and relationships—including his relationship with you.

- Emphasize the processes he is involved in, not only the

goals—the game, not the score. The worst basketball or baseball player can have the best time if he is not handicapped by self-conscious performance anxiety. Trying his best should be rewarded as fully as being the best.

- Reinforce mastery, not competition. Fixing cars, fixing clocks, or fixing computers involves skills that are fun to exercise. Curiosity seems to be an inborn drive, but you must also nurture it in your child.

- Remember the leave/return pattern of separation, and let him return when he is frightened. If you fear that his leaving means he'll never come back, or that his coming back means he'll never try to leave again, you may be conveying this anxiety and setting up a self-fulfilling prophecy (as in the case of Ron and his mother). Both Olga Silverstein of the Ackerman Family Institute and psychiatrist John Bowlby agree that the mother is most important here. She must let the child know that she supports his move toward autonomy and that she is still there if he needs her.

- Encourage his nurturing instincts. You don't have to take away his football, or his motorized space station, but you might add a stuffed animal if he is young or a babysitting job if he is older. Studies show that the father is most important here. He must let his son know that real men can hug their boy as well as hit a baseball.

TURBULENT TEENS AND TESTOSTERONE

"Puberty" is a term that refers to the *physical* development between childhood and adulthood. For some, body changes are gradual as their shape becomes adult; for others, many growth spurts take them by surprise.

"Adolescence" is a term that refers to the *psychological* development between "childhood" and "adulthood." For some, this corresponds to the teen years, while for others it extends into their twenties. The average teen has to cope with the stresses of both adolescence and puberty.

Puberty usually begins at about twelve years and peaks at thirteen to fourteen years; but it can begin as early as ten or as late as sixteen or seventeen. Two hormones are produced by the hypothalamus in the brain, and they in turn stimulate the testes to produce sperm and to produce the male hormone testosterone. The production of sperm means that the boy can now become a biological father. The testosterone means that his pubic hair will grow, his penis will grow, his length and strength will grow, his mustache will grow, and last but not least, his self-consciousness will grow (particularly if he is a late or early starter).

Even if he is right on time in his development, the teen's tolerance for change is tested. Never again will so much change so quickly:

1. The preteen is a compact, well-coordinated package. At puberty, however, different parts of the body start to grow at different rates, a process that is called "dysynchrony," and which feels like disaster.

2. The activity of glands produces strong body odor and acne for the first time—at just the wrong time!

3. As testosterone increases, so does the frequency of spontaneous erections, wet dreams, and morning erections. The average teen is embarrassed by the first, surprised by the second, and misinformed about the third (morning erections have nothing to do with full bladders), and he also tends to be guilt-ridden by his interest in masturbation.

4. Many boys have temporary breast swelling when they begin puberty. If they are overweight, this will be more pronounced and will compound self-consciousness.

5. Teen growth seems to be never-ending. In fact, many

boys keep growing until they are in their twenties! That's a long time to wait before they see how they are going to turn out.

6. Voice changes are rarely smooth. As the larynx enlarges, the male's voice deepens—but not without months of squeaks and cracks.

Adolescence includes puberty but ends with psychological adulthood, not physical maturity. If this strikes you as vague, it is. Adulthood involves emotional, financial, and/or residential independence, and for some the period of adolescence may be very long indeed. It also means that adolescence will be a time when the boy must learn to deal with the stresses that accompany this maturation, or he will not be able to move on. Some men never do, and psychologist Dan Kiley termed this the "Peter Pan Syndrome." Those men who do move on beyond adolescence must first deal with the following stresses.

SEXUAL STRESS

Through adolescence, girls are generally more advanced physically and socially than boys. The boys, however, are more often telling each other about their sexual successes. Interestingly enough, my male patients tell me that the torture of anticipating rejection when they were young was second only to the torture of anticipating acceptance. If a girl rejected their advances, they felt like fools and usually lied to their friends. If a girl accepted their advances, they felt like fools and often ejaculated prematurely or acted immaturely. And again, control became an important issue.

Despite the sexual revolution, the average age of first intercourse for young men today is about the same as it was in their grandfather's time a half-century ago: between sixteen and nineteen years old. The rates of venereal disease, however, have not stayed the same, despite sex education in school. The rates of sexually transmitted diseases (STDs) have soared—in part because the pill doesn't provide the same degree of protection against disease, for either the man or the woman, that the condom does; in part because young women who are sexually active are less realistic about STDs than older women; in part because there is more sexual activity among teenagers in general; and in part because, many surveys suggest, teenagers believe they will either be lucky or that such diseases, except for AIDS, are easily cured.

Myths about the male of the species abound during this period, creating unnecessary stress in already-stressed adolescents. Many young men believe that they can "use up" their virility temporarily or permanently by masturbating or being too sexually active. Others believe that they will lose their capacity for erection if they *don't* make frequent use of it. Most young men believe that their partners are going to judge them on performance rather than pleasure. Unfortunately, this means that they will become very orgasm-focused, and that hugging, petting, and foreplay become moments of anxious anticipation rather than activities enjoyable in themselves. As he gets older, the young man will have little practice taking in the stimulation he will need to respond with an erection.

The best antidote to myths is information: if you are a young man and confused about the facts in this area, seek to learn as much as you can; if you are a parent whose son may be confused, help him get the information he needs.

SCHOOL STRESS

Some boys are concerned about getting into college, some about vocational choice, some about pleasing their parents with high grades, some about hiding high grades from "the guys," some about bringing up low grades, some about earning a living while they are in high school. All these things and more can contribute to school stress—and almost every boy has some of it.

After I appeared on a television program in Baltimore, Maryland, three teenage boys visited me in the studio. They had heard me talking on the air about stress management, and raced to catch me before the show ended. A schoolmate had just committed suicide the week before, and they wanted to give me a message to make public to parents in general. "Let parents know," they said, "that the pressure to please them with good grades can get to be too much. Sometimes we just can't do it because we're not as smart as they'd like us to be. We think that's why our friend committed suicide," they said.

Actually, statistics show that suicide victims among college students are more likely to have higher than lower grades. This does not mean, however, that they are not under academic pressure. In fact, these may be the very boys who are most sensitive to academic pressure, who try harder and succeed more, but who rate their achievements lower. Among high school students, poor grades, truancy, expulsion, learning difficulties, classroom disruption, and/or excessive concern about school pressure are often part of the high-risk suicide profile.

In addition, according to Alan Berman at the Washington Psychological Center, most suicidal teens had suffered from an "inordinate amount of stress within the preceding twelve months and a home broken by divorce, remarriage, or marital discord." Although teenage girls are more likely than teenage boys to attempt suicide as "cries for help," boys are more likely to succeed when they try it. In 1990, the suicide death rate of teenage boys was four times higher than that of teenage girls. The rate for white teenage boys was about one and a half times higher than that of black teenage boys. Male teens, like adult men, commit suicide violently, using guns or explosives, or hanging themselves.

FAMILY STRESS

Family problems are the number-one reason for admission to day hospitals, for calls placed to telephone hot lines, and for visits to emergency services in the United States. Sometimes the family problems center around the teen, sometimes not. Either way, family discord creates stress for teens struggling to understand their role in the home, at school, and in the outside world.

The teenage boy is often the center of a family problem if the mother, father, or even live-in grandparents are arguing about rules, regulations, and responsibilities for the young man. Some families expect their sons to contribute money to the household budget, some do not. Some families expect their sons to participate within the family time and recreation structure, some do not. Some families expect their sons to follow the family's own traditional career and life-style patterns, some do not. There is no single scenario that works for every family, but there is definitely one that never works: parents openly disagreeing with each other about everything, including what is expected of their son. If parents keep changing the rules or sabotaging each other's messages to their son, this emotional flux added to the already numerous bodily, social, and academic changes that the teen is experiencing will likely overwhelm him.

It is often said that the mother helps the child learn how to live within the home, and the father helps the child learn to move out into the world. The mother, then, nurtures emotional bonding, and the father nurtures emotional independence. If the teenage boy experiences continual conflict between his parents, he's not likely to be learning either lesson. Furthermore, it also interferes with his successful identification with a male role model. To move from being "a kid" to being "a man," the teenage boy looks for a man to emulate—usually his father. He wants his father to be strong, protective, and important. He wants his father to resolve conflicts by prevailing over his mother or grandmother, and may even bring conflicts to a head to force his father's hand.

Calls from school counselors, frequent accidents, distracted or disorganized behavior, and delinquency can all be signs of a boy's seeming inability to deal with stress in the outside world. "See," he might be saying, "I'm like you, Dad; real men are always in the middle of conflict." He might secretly *want* to say, "Show me how to cope without all this conflict."

Although parents may try to hide family problems that do not directly involve their teenage boy, he will soon pick up clues in their behavior that something is wrong. The mystery of a parent's illness, financial reverses, or potential separation or divorce is usually harder for the teen to deal with than the reality. Sharing information, though not necessarily details, with him may help. This is one way of saying that he is seen by you as emerging emotionally and that there is nothing "too terrible" to talk about.

SEPARATION STRESS

The process of separation from the primary family, which started during the preteen years, continues during the teenage years. By nineteen, many men are living away from home: at college, in the military, married, or supporting their own apartment. Many others are still living at home but trying to feel separated, nonetheless. They have been asked, "What do you want to be when you grow up?" since they were toddlers, and now they must begin to find out. They have been prepared for being "their own men" since they were boys, and now it's time to do it. They have been warned that "It's a cruel world out there," and now they must face this truth.

One way to separate emotionally from one's father is to begin to challenge him and compete with him. A boy's first image of his father was created long ago. Daddy was usually seen as big and strong and powerful. It tends to be that first image, not the current reality, that teenagers are emulating and trying to surpass. This produces several potential stresses:

1. If the young man feels that he has surpassed his father, then he must continue on without a "father figure" to emulate. This may make him feel angry and alone.

2. If the young man remains in competition with his father, then he has not really separated from his father at all. Instead he has maintained a very involved connection and father-focus.

3. If the young man liked being "Daddy's little boy," then he may have to go away angry if he is to go away at all.

He may have to hang on to all the negatives about home to make it possible for him to leave. He may even have to create problems to make home seem less inviting and dependency less enticing.

A boy raised without a father may have a special problem during this period of separation. Although his friends may be important to his social life and may influence his style of dress and language, a teenager's political, religious, and vocational opinions more often follow those of his father. Without a father in the home, a teenage boy is on his own in these areas. Identifying with his mother's positions may make him fearful that he is thinking like a woman and may create an identity confusion. In addition, a teenage boy often uses his father not only to emulate, but to rebel against. He may want to test his capacity for independence by temporarily rejecting his father and trying to survive financially or psychologically without him. If there is no father, there is no opportunity to test himself in this way.

Big brothers, uncles, stepfathers, and some mothers can help a boy learn to separate if they understand the father's role—that is, not to mold the boy, but to provide a model. If the father accepts himself, the teenage boy is likely to do the same. If the father is flexible and understanding, the boy is also likely to be. If the father is absent, then this fathering must be provided by others.

The teenage boy must also deal with separation from his mother—his first true love. By the time most boys are four, they have "proposed" to their mothers. By the time they are fourteen, they have fallen in love with someone else! One way to separate from one's mother, then, is to bond with a girlfriend. She may be practicing the mother-wife role herself, which suits a teenage male very well. Too often, however, teens reach for a separate identity by marrying—they substitute marriage for adulthood and switch their identity from "son" to "husband" and even "father" to prove their independence.

Another way a boy can force himself away from the comforting arms of childhood is to join the military or any organization that takes over the family function. These organizations each provide structure, leadership, rules, companionship, and rewards. They give their members an identity, and can help give teens a sense of separation from their families. But these organizations just put off for a while a real confrontation with the world. In fact, if they require emotional channeling, conformity, or competitiveness, they may be slowing down a boy's movement toward an individual sense of responsibility and accountability.

SELF-AWARENESS STRESS

Teenage girls are not alone in their preoccupation with their appearances. Boys are acutely aware of themselves, too. Acne, glasses, ears too big, height too short, skinny, heavy, buck teeth, braces, warts, long necks, wide feet . . . just part of the package deal to adults, but significant sources of stress to teenage boys. Men who participated in the Male Stress Survey remember feeling that they were being punished for an unknown failure or inadequacy when they looked in the mirror and saw flaws. Many worked on body building to build up not only their muscles but also their sense of control over their appearances and their bodies. It helped them feel that they could protect themselves, physically and emotionally. No matter how they felt inside, outside they looked strong!

Questions of life and death, of values, God, morality, and man's meaning also occupy and preoccupy the thoughts of many teenagers.

Steve remembers lying in bed as a teen and thinking. "I was thinking about the size of the universe, the size of me, and about death. I was thinking about being dead forever, and suddenly I couldn't stand it. I was terrified. I went into the kitchen and put the light on. My father must have been up, because in a few minutes he came out and asked me what was wrong. I told him and asked what he thought about death and eternity and life after death. He seemed very sad. He said he'd been thinking about it for a long time and still didn't have any answers. We talked some more and then I went to bed again. That was about ten years ago, and I've only just now understood that he couldn't give me any other answer because he couldn't bring himself to lie. But for a long time, I wished he *had* lied. I wished he could tell me something nice and comforting whether he believed it or not."

Teenagers often rethink answers learned years before in religion class or at home to see if the explanations still suit them. Sometimes they decide that these do. Sometimes they search for their own answers and may even come to the same conclusions that their parents did. Often they find different perspectives, perhaps to reaffirm their developing independence. The process is stressful, though important, because these questions cannot be answered for many teens in absolute terms.

WORLD-AWARENESS STRESS

Teens test not only early answers to questions about life and death, but also political and social answers to questions about daily life. They are exposed to the world community through radio, television, and newspapers. They have an increased awareness of the world's threats, deficiencies, and opportunities. They are sharply aware of water and air pollution, and what it may do to their bodies. They often know a good deal about nuclear weapons and nuclear energy controversies, and what the outcomes may mean for themselves and their children. They are, in general, aware of the imperfections of society, and know three facts:

1. As teens they are quite powerless to change the world community.
2. There are no simple answers.
3. Someday soon *they* will be the adults and will have to assume responsibility for their own world and the world community.

TEEN MALE STRESS SYMPTOMS

Some stress symptoms suffered by teens are shared by adult men: smoking, overeating, irritability, depression, disorganization, decision-making problems, and dependency feelings. But teenagers are also subject to more serious symptoms: accidents, substance abuse, and antisocial behavior.

ACCIDENTS

Just as adults become more vulnerable to accidents under stress, so do teenagers. R. Dean Coddington and Jeffrey R. Troxell studied 114 high-school football players and found that those who had experienced more family instability were more likely to sustain significant injuries. The types of instability singled out as especially stressful were parental illness, separation, divorce, and death. The leading cause of death among fifteen- to twenty-four-year-old white males is accidents. Teenage boys are more likely to die from gunshot wounds than from all natural causes combined.

In *Coping with Teenage Depression,* Kathleen McCoy reports that many studies link injuries and car accidents to teen depression. Why is the rate of both injuries and car accidents higher for boys? Probably because risk-taking lifts them from their depression in an acceptable "macho" manner, whereas crying or talking about their feelings would make them feel embarrassed. Their risks lead them toward accidents or may even be veiled suicide attempts, attention-getting behavior that turns out to be more self-destructive than successful.

SUBSTANCE ABUSE

Alcohol and drug abuse are not confined to teenage males, but the incidence of both is growing among teens. Although parents are usually less alarmed about their sons' drinking than about their using drugs, alcohol is a "liquid barbiturate" that is potent and addictive. Annual national surveys of 17,000 high-school seniors show that alcohol is by far the drug most used by this group and male college students and young adults tend to drink substantially more than females. In 1990, for example, 90 percent said they had tried alcohol and 32 percent reported heavy drinking (five or more drinks in a row) during the two weeks prior to the survey interview. This is alarming in that alcohol not only disinhibits antisocial behavior, affects memory, and does damage to the body, but it also slows motor reflexes and interferes with visual motor coordination. In other words, alcohol is contributing to the enormous number of male teenage deaths from car accidents. This drug may reduce teen stress for the moment, but only increases the stress syndrome ultimately by adding yet another area that the teenage male feels is beyond his control.

Boys are not only three times more likely than girls to become alcohol-dependent, they are also 50 percent more likely to use illicit drugs. Marijuana is the second most frequently used drug by teenagers (27 percent). Although availability is the most significant determinant of drug use, it is stress that can determine which drug or how much of a given drug will be used.

In fact, a study by A. Vaux and M. Ruggiero correlates both drug abuse and juvenile delinquency with the stresses of life changes. Think of teen drug abuse as an attempt at self-medication. Agitated teens will reach for sedative-hypnotics like alcohol, barbiturates, tranquilizers, and "downers." Depressed teens will reach for amphetamines, cocaine, nicotine, and other "uppers." Disenchanted and overwhelmed teens will reach for hallucinogenics like marijuana, LSD, and hashish, or narcotics like heroin, in order to alter their minds or create a state of euphoria. Such stress escapes mean time-out, however, from psychological growth as well. The teen is then left having to face his original stresses, plus his new dependency, plus physical or psychological damage, plus lost time.

ANTI-SOCIAL BEHAVIOR

After reviewing dozens of studies, Bruce E. Compas of the

University of Vermont concluded that the accumulated evidence definitely supports the notion that stressful life events in childhood are associated with psychological and behavioral problems. In fact, according to Compas, chronic strains and daily stressors play a greater role than major life events in the development of psychological and behavioral problems during adolescence. In any case, the greater the amount of either change or daily stress a boy must cope with, the greater his chances of antisocial behavior. It makes sense, then, that the more there is overcrowding, family discord, lack of affection, inconsistency, or neglect, the more likely the boy will be delinquent. The extent to which delinquency can be seen as a teenage male stress symptom is reflected in the following information about teenagers eighteen and under from the U.S. Federal Bureau of Investigation's *Crimes in the United States*, 1992.

- Over ten times more boys than girls were arrested for robbery.

- Five times more boys than girls were arrested for assault.

- Ten times more boys than girls were arrested for burglary.

- As for motor vehicle theft, more than seven times more boys were arrested than girls.

- Almost ten times more boys than girls were arrested for arson.

- Fifteen times more boys than girls were arrested for sex offenses.

- For disorderly conduct, close to four times more boys were arrested than girls.

- As for "driving under the influence" (which includes alcohol and drugs), ten times as many boys were arrested as girls.

It is likely that many factors combine to make delinquent

behavior a teenage male stress symptom, rather than a female one.

1. Boys may have more opportunity for night behavior, since they are often given more freedom and independence than girls of the same age.

2. Boys may be trying to counteract depression by engaging in daredevil behavior and risk-taking, whereas girls typically handle depression differently (for example, through eating disturbances such as anorexia and bulimia).

3. Boys may be testing parental limits and love in this way. In their anxiety about the "worst that could happen to them if they were on their own," they may be trying to make the worst come true while their parents are still around to bail them out—or seeing if they will still be loved if they fail out there.

4. Boys may be defying police authority in a symbolic defiance of their fathers. Whereas teenage girls tend to go through a period of estrangement from their mothers, teen boys often feel estranged from their fathers. Writer Mark Twain pointed out that when he was fourteen his father knew nothing, but when he was twenty-one he was amazed at how much the old man had learned in seven years!

5. Boys may be expressing the violence that they learned was "manly" behavior through media messages. Reality and fantasy are often not clearly differentiated for young teens or disturbed young adults. If a teenage boy is trying to get attention or punish his parents through his embarrassing behavior, the six o'clock news will show him that violence gets national attention.

TEEN STRESS MANAGEMENT

Adolescence is a time of turbulence for parents as well as their teenagers. To help both yourself and your son cope, study the stress management techniques outlined in Chapter 9 and practice them whenever possible. Unless your son needs professional help because he is showing one of the more serious stress symptoms discussed, your own fresh look at the situation—your own sense of perspective—can also help ease a lot of the tension.

Examine your attitude toward your son, especially toward the issue of control. Are you treating him more as a preteenager than an adolescent; does he deserve more autonomy than you've given him? Then change your attitude, if necessary.

Treat your reasonable expectations as being reasonable. It's reasonable to expect a fourteen-year-old boy to keep his room moderately neat most of the time. But don't *ask* if he's done it when you know he hasn't, because this feels like a manipulation. It's better to come out plainly with something like, "I see you haven't fixed your room yet and I'd like you to do it."

As I've noted, adolescence is a time when your son starts to feel a very strong need to achieve, and it's common for parents to feel that same need with him: if the son doesn't make a straight-A average, the parents have failed. Give yourself and your son permission not to be perfect, not to be Superman, Superwoman, and Superboy. If he needs help, see that he gets it, but don't make him live up to your ideals and increase the pressure (on you and on him) if he seems to be "failing." Instead, give him permission to find his own ideals and help him reach them.

Finally, practice. Practice talking to each other, practice resolving problems by discussing them. The results can last a lifetime. E. C. Burnett, Jr., showed that young adults raised in families who settled problems nonviolently were able to handle conflicts much better than young adults from violent families ("violence" being defined as at least two violent incidents in ten years). The main alternative to violence is talking, and that's also the best defense against stress.

Practice setting reasonable limits and sticking to them. Teenagers need limits because they are still learning how to be adults. Teenagers need limits because they want to feel that their parents are still watching over them. Teenagers need limits so that they can test them. If you don't set reasonable limits for them, teenagers will push you into doing so with outrageous, self-destructive, or attention-getting behaviors. Don't be afraid to fight the small battles over curfews and grades. They may save you from the larger battles concerning drugs and dropping out. They are likely to inspire your teenager's respect.

Practice flexibility. Haim Ginot spelled out two criteria for permissiveness in his book *Between Parent and Child:*

1. Allow leeway for learners. A driver with a learner's permit, Dr. Ginot points out, is not given a ticket when he signals right and turns left. The learner is clearly moving toward future improvement. A teenager can be viewed as an adult-in-training. As long as he is moving in that direction, allow for mistakes.

2. Allow leeway for hard times. Recognize high stress periods and expect disrupted or unusual behavior. A teenager who has just moved, who is coping with his parents' divorce, whose best friend has died, or who has been ill is more likely to be irritable or withdrawn, distracted or defiant.

And, above all, practice keeping your sense of humor. If you can laugh at yourself, your teenage son will learn to laugh with you and at himself. Things are rarely as hopeless as they can seem to a teenager under stress.

6 HIDDEN STRESSES

IT'S BEEN A HARD DAY, BUT YOU ARE NOT TOO SURE WHY. YOU FEEL IRRI-
tated, worn down, impatient, and tired. You'd like to have an
excuse to argue, yell, or storm out of the house in a grand exit,
but no one at home is starting up with you. Why do you feel this
way when you haven't been fired, side-swiped, or mugged?

Ask your wife, your daughter, or your mother. The hundreds
of women I surveyed about male stress noticed that their
fathers, sons, and mates are often pushed into stress symptoms
by situations that are not *obviously* stressful. Call these the hidden stresses; they each appeared again and again on the lists of
male stresses compiled by women. They each brought a smile
or a grimace of recognition to the faces of the men interviewed
for this book. They may be silent and subtle, but they are prime
contributors to the Male Stress Syndrome nonetheless!

HIDDEN STRESS #1: CHANGES IN ROUTINE

Big changes are obviously stressful: a new baby, a different
job, a new house, an illness, a divorce, a retirement. Small

changes in routine are less obviously stressful, but make their impact felt just the same: a commute being rerouted, a desk being moved, a favorite diner closing, a diet commencing, a coffee break being eliminated, a program being preempted, a privilege being taken away.

Sometimes changes in routine foreshadow larger changes that are just beginning. Sometimes they interfere with rituals that are very comforting during times of flux. Sometimes they force a reexamination of daily satisfactions and dissatisfactions. Sometimes they result in an inconvenience that sounds minor but feels major. Sometimes they undermine a sense of control. Sometimes they even undermine a sense of identity.

> Sam was a top graphics man, but all his firm could give him when he started there was the most battered drafting board in the world. Scratches, nicks, gouges, gashes, paint splotches—according to his wife, this board had had it. It bothered her, but didn't seem to bother Sam. The firm eventually ordered a new board for Sam and when it came he thanked them warmly. In the office he acted as if he appreciated the new board. At home, he complained that he couldn't get into his work that week, that he had trouble falling asleep and found he awakened early. After he had spent some extra time in the office, however, things seemed to get better. Some weeks later, on her next visit to the office for lunch with Sam, his wife noticed that his new board now looked just like his old board.

Here are some suggestions for counteracting Hidden Stress #1 from a chief executive officer (CEO) who changed companies after twenty years.

- Try to leave your breakfast rituals intact; start the day with stability. Toast at home, tea at the diner, or coffee at your desk can help you feel like you are starting the day *your* way.

- Take over the new routine and make it "yours" as quickly as you can. Find its advantages and take the new change one step further. This can help you regain a sense of choice and control—and save you from wasting energy on resistance or feeling resentment about complying.

HIDDEN STRESS #2: SOCIAL ANXIETY

They attend conventions and cocktail parties, and join pick-up touch-football games, but most men are somewhat anxious anticipating new situations such as these. Warren Jones of the University of Tulsa and Dan Russell of the University of Ohio College of Medicine list the following hidden social stresses that men expect themselves to handle with no problem, but which often give them trouble. Review the list yourself and check those that apply to you. The key here is that men have learned that they "should not" be anxious in these situations, but are anxious anyway. Women, on the other hand, often expect themselves to be nervous in these situations, and are surprised when they are not!

_____ parties with strangers

_____ giving speeches

_____ answering personal questions in public

_____ meeting a date's parents

_____ first day on a new job

_____ being the butt of a practical joke

_____ talking with someone in authority

_____ going on a job interview

_____ attending a formal dinner party

_____ handling a blind date

Three-quarters of the hundreds of people interviewed by Jones and Russell admitted to being stressed at parties with strangers and dreaded having to give a speech. Even down at the bottom of the list, more than 40 percent of the study group were nervous about blind dates, and almost 60 percent worried about meeting their date's parents.

Some symptoms of this hidden stress?

1. Negative thoughts: "Here's where I make a fool of myself."

2. Negative self-evaluation, no matter how well you actually did: "I made a fool of myself."

3. Exaggerating or focusing on the negative evaluations of others, ignoring or forgetting the positive feedback: "I'm always making a fool of myself, and now everyone knows it."

4. Crediting your successes to external factors and your failures to yourself: "I lucked out this time, but basically I'm a fool."

If you recognize these symptoms of social anxiety, it is time to switch your focus from watching yourself through others' eyes to concentrating on what those around you are doing. Watching yourself will increase your anxiety. Looking at others should increase your social curiosity, information, and involvement, instead. In fact, you may find that others are more concerned with your approval of *them* than with their approval of *you*!

HIDDEN STRESS #3: FEAR OF FAILURE

Most men will rate their need for achievement higher than their fear of failure, but their behavior may be saying something different. Picture this: You are participating in a ring-toss game, and you are told that you may stand as close as you would like to the stake—or as far away. If you know that you would walk right up to the stake and drop the rings over it from above, fear of failure is probably not one of your hidden stresses. But if you picture yourself moving back from the stake to make the task more "challenging," then you are probably providing yourself with an excuse for failure under the guise of increasing the value of achievement.

Gary had been offered the opportunity of a lifetime. He had a small printing business that supplied personalized stationery to retail shops for their customers and to the local Board of Education. Now he was being offered the opportunity to become the supplier for the entire county government. Gary had the know-how, skill, and equipment. But he didn't have the perspective. He knew the retailers and the members of the local Board of Education personally, and he felt comfortable explaining delays or errors to them. He didn't know the county executive or her staff personally, and feared that he might be seen as incompetent if he made an error. Gary became so focused on his imaginary embarrassment should he ever fail in this larger arena that he stepped out of the arena altogether, telling them that the job was "too big" for his operation. Gary felt avoiding failure was in his best interest.

What about the fun of success? What about the reality that everyone makes mistakes? Just think of the number of times you may be unknowingly handicapping yourself and making your life more stressed because of concern about the opinions of others. Failure means shame, not simple disappointment, so excuses must always be handy.

- Do you procrastinate so that you can always say that "too little time" kept you from doing better?
- Do you overschedule yourself so that you can always say that "too much to do" is your problem?
- Do you take the roundabout or difficult route to your goals, so that your fear of failure will be hidden by the fight to overcome overwhelming odds?
- Do you avoid attractive women because they may turn you down?
- Do you rule yourself out of a promotion application because you may be passed over?
- Do you say to yourself that it is better not to try than to try and not succeed?

If so, fear of failure is contributing to your Male Stress Syndrome. Reducing fear-of-failure behavior begins with recognition. Try to catch yourself in the process of backing away from a goal or "spectatoring," looking at yourself through others' eyes (for more on spectatoring, see Hidden Stress #7). Then reassess the situation from a new point of view: your *aims*, not your aim. Concentrate on what you want to accomplish, not what you think others think you should accomplish. Finally, make yourself try the simple, direct approach. If you succeed, give yourself credit. If you fail, allow yourself disappointment, not disapproval. After all, why add your own insults to injury?

HIDDEN STRESS #4: CONTROL OF CHILDREN

Many men say they worry about their children in general, but it's their wives and mothers who pinpoint the stress more precisely. They notice that as children become more autonomous and independent, fathers become more anxious about the relationship. Most men seem to be relatively calm about the toddler's crying, schoolyard fights, or run-of-the-mill childhood illness. It is their child's first date, career decisions, marriage, or move to a far-off location that worries them.

The reasons are many. Control over children is in fact diminished as children mature and become financially and psychologically independent. As we've seen, reduced control usually means increased stress. For many fathers, this is also associated with a concern that they can no longer protect their children from life's realities. This can mean a loss of position since much of fathering involves providing and protecting.

One answer to this problem is to try fathering without the need to be a father figure. Let yourself become a person to your child; offer your advice and opinions, but resist the need to have your child follow your way. The more your growing children resist your control, the more likely it is that you are either trying to overregulate their lives, or that you personalize their decisions too much. There are often many scripts for the same scenario. Don't think their decisions must be the same as those you would have made in their place. Try to hear them as separate people whom you love, not mere reflections of yourself. And only *think*, never say unless you're asked, "When I was your age...."

HIDDEN STRESS #5:
CONTROL OF CIRCUMSTANCES

Men and women alike experience increased stress when they feel a situation is beyond their control, but because of their early training men tend to interpret a greater number of situations as "control" situations, and they react more dramatically to them. For example:

- Men are stressed when they are forced to be in the passenger seat rather than at the wheel of an automobile.

- Men are stressed when they must wait for a table at a restaurant, or on line for a movie, and they frequently choose to forgo the meal or movie to regain their sense of choice.

- Men become irate at gridlock, infuriated by road construction, and exasperated at "stupid" drivers who distract or detain them.

- Men dread funerals and psychotherapy, and sometimes equate the two as depressing reminders of life's uncertainties.

- Men postpone dental appointments and other procedures that require that they put themselves in others' hands.

- Men are terrified of illness or injury that may interfere with their ability to be in charge of their daily lives.

- Men prefer requests to demands, and free choice to requests—and they will demonstrate this by saying "no" to suggestions for things that they might actually have enjoyed.

I call this particular hidden stress *circumstantial claustrophobia.* If a man feels locked into a situation, his focus often shifts from whether or not the situation suits him to whether or not he feels that he has a choice about it. "Will you marry me?"

is a proposal if a man asks; it is pressure if a woman asks! "Kiss me" is assertive on his lips, aggressive on hers.

Since real life inevitably brings situations beyond our control, management of the Male Stress Syndrome must include the ability to *give up the struggle for control* when that struggle is unrealistic. Assess your chances of changing a situation before you invest your adrenaline. Even more important, assess how desirable a situation really might be before you fight it or flee from it—you may choose to relish rather than relinquish it.

HIDDEN STRESS #6: COMMITMENT CODES

Every day in every way, a man defines himself in terms of his word. He has learned that his word is his honor, and that he is only as good as his word. With every type of personal communication, then, comes a certain amount of male stress. Every appointment becomes a commitment. Every promise becomes a test of character. Every offer becomes an oath.

The Male Stress Survey asked men to complete the sentence: "When I try to make a personal commitment, I ——————." Their answers confirm the strength of the commitment code among men:

"I do it at all costs."
"I hold up my end."
"I try my best and more."
"I do what is *right*."
"I feel guilty if I don't follow through."
"I overdo it."
"I never change my mind."
"I finish it."
"I must do it."

These answers were consistent for men of all ages (eighteen

to seventy-nine years) and across all socioeconomic and education levels. They throw an interesting light on the common observation that the man of the nineties has a "commitment problem." It seems that male stress comes not from an inability to make commitments, but from the pressure men put on themselves once the commitment is made. If, in fact, you have learned that your word is a promise and that a promise is a pact, then holding back from making commitments would be a way of managing stress levels.

Unfortunately, holding back from making commitments may create even more stress in the long run. Weekend plans, potential business deals, and even marriage partners may be lost forever because of an overinvestment in "the word." A more practical defense against this male stress would involve building option clauses and appropriate contingency alternatives into your consents and commitments. "I am willing to try" might replace "Let's do it." "I'll do my best to make this work" might replace "I'll make it happen."

HIDDEN STRESS #7: SPECTATORING

The term "spectatoring" first arose in sex therapy, with men who were worried about impotence. During foreplay, they kept checking up on the state of their erections, to see how they were doing. This very act, this spectatoring, practically guaranteed that they would have erectile problems.

Spectatoring, then, is checking up on your performance *while you are in the middle of it,* not after. It is the tennis player wondering if he's holding the racket at the proper angle. It is the sales director, in the middle of a talk, wondering if the sound of his voice is authoritative. It is the accountant wondering if he is adding the figures correctly, losing his place, and having to start again. It is the young man wondering, in the middle of the disco, whether he looks awkward—and then losing the beat.

Spectatoring is not only a symptom of male stress, but a cause as well. To avoid criticism by their parents, peers, or partners, men learn to criticize themselves first, to beat everyone else to the punch and appear near-perfect. Many women say that they do this in particular situations; men seem to do it more constantly. There is a constant vigilance that many men feel must accompany their performances with their family, on the job, or in bed. It is a cause of stress because it interferes with behavior that could be spontaneous and natural. Activities that might otherwise be stress-reducing, like sex, sports, or socializing, now become forced and artificial.

Women complain that men's spectatoring creates a hidden stress for them, also. They point out that a man preoccupied with his own "performance" is out of touch with others. Wives, lovers, and friends become an audience to worry about, rather than people to interact with and listen to. Pleasure is lost, and stress is increased, for both. If you catch yourself spectatoring, practice refocusing on the information coming in to you, rather than on the information you believe *others* think you are giving out.

During sex, for example, focus on the touch of your partner's hand and tell her when she is making you feel good. If you find your thoughts wandering to a concern about her being bored or tired or deprived, mention your concern. If she reassures you, refocus on the pleasure that she is giving you. She will definitely not be bored if she sees that she is having a positive effect on you!

During a speech, for example, remain focused on what you want to say to your audience, not on what your audience might want to say to you. Until mental telepathy is perfected, you'll never really know, anyway. So wait until the question-and-answer period to deal with their thoughts. Until then, give them yours to deal with.

During a dance, for example, check out how you feel, not how you think you look. Ask yourself if you are having fun, not whether you are unwittingly providing entertainment. Remember, everyone else is probably too worried about themselves or enjoying themselves too much to really be focused on *your* performance.

HIDDEN STRESS #8: AUTHORITY ANXIETY

A true authoritarian personality takes orders as readily as he gives them. He is comfortable with the concept of a chain of command and is committed to following orders and weeding out weak links in the chain. He can take responsibility for those beneath him, but is also willing to turn over responsibility for his own actions to those above him in rank or power. Most American men are *not* true authoritarian personalities!

This is both good news and bad news. It's good news that American men are not raised to submit to a "Big Brother" mentality. They're better at giving orders than taking them; they exercise their freedom of speech and tend to hold themselves accountable for their own actions. It's bad news, though, in those special circumstances where men must interact with blind authority, bureaucratic red tape, or military mandates. Such interactions usually create male stress in its most intense forms.

A man is taught to act fast, take charge, be autonomous, and feel responsible, but he is often put in positions of subservience or submission. His adrenaline prepares him for fight or flight, but neither tactic is effective. When legalities overrule logic, when common sense yields to common practice, his aggressive impulses often begin to overflow with nowhere to go. Fear of such a loss of control over impulses is called anxiety. I call this particular male stress "authority anxiety."

Authority anxiety can sneak up on you at any moment. The bus driver who arbitrarily decides to skip a stop, the waiter who behaves as if he owns the diner, the secretary who will not put your call through, the traffic cop who is ignoring eastbound cars, the boss who decrees impossible deadlines, and the federal employee who does paperwork while people wait all evoke this stress. Everything a man has been taught about channeling emotions, controlling himself, and performing effectively is being tested. He is not being seen or heard.

To manage this male stress there is one major rule: *Do not personalize the situation.* It may be infuriating, but don't perceive it as insulting. It may be inane, but it doesn't mean *you* should act insane. Look for the best angle of approach, and the most effective avenue of action—not for the momentary relief of an emotional explosion or the debilitating effects of an inner fury. If a desk clerk cannot find your reservation, don't react; ask him to *act.* Put him in charge and tell him you are confident that he can rectify the situation. If your wife is not listening to your explanation or believing your truthful story, ask her what she would like to hear. In cases of authority anxiety, in other words, defensiveness is the worst defense.

HIDDEN STRESS #9: FATHER'S DEATH

The death of parents is not by any means a "hidden" stress. It is a stress that is universally recognized and provided for by religious and social customs and mourning rituals. The special meaning of a father's death to a man, however, is not always obvious to him.

It had been a year since Jeffrey's father died, but he was still feeling its effects. He had been strong for his mother and his children during the funeral and the weeks following. He had been available for the lawyers and accountants working on the estate problems in the months afterward. He had known his father's death was coming for a year before. But he was unprepared for the feelings that began six months later. He realized that he was no longer "the kid." To his father, and to himself, while his father was alive, he had always been "the kid." When his father died he ceased being his father's son and became his own son's father. He was now the oldest male in his family—and he feared his own mortality. The world at large seemed changed; his world certainly was.

As in the case of Jeffrey, men often feel young while their father lives. When he dies, there is a generational shift and the son joins the "older" generation. This can evoke concerns associated with aging, illness, responsibility, and even death. The son is often now in charge of his mother's well-being; he must step into his father's shoes.

Stepping into his father's shoes has other meanings as well. If he does not fill his father's shoes yet in terms of achievement, income, or prestige, the experience can make him feel inadequate and stressed. If he has already outgrown his father's shoes, on the other hand, he may feel angry that his father did not leave a more impressive social legacy. If he is about to grow in his career, he may feel acute disappointment that his father will not be alive to applaud his success. If he was competitive with his father, as most sons are to some extent, then he likely feels cheated out of a sense of potential victory.

Recognizing that all these feelings are normal can help reduce the surprise and guilt that surround them. As a man begins to parent himself, his stress usually subsides and is replaced by acceptance. His father may become gradually more, rather than less, vivid in his memory, and he may come to feel like a son and a father simultaneously.

HIDDEN STRESS #10: FEMALE STRESS

"Men can fix anything except feelings," complained one woman whose partner was filling out the Male Stress Survey form. He joined us, and agreed. "When Donna becomes tearful or fearful, I become more upset than she is." Why? "Because I feel that I have to make things right. When I can't, I feel frustrated. When I can't, I feel as though I've failed her."

Most men agreed with Donna's husband. They said they had learned all their lives that they were expected to solve problems by taking action. When the problem was not theirs, taking action was not usually appropriate or helpful or even possible. As Donald Bell, a Harvard professor of social history, explained the problem in his book *Being a Man,* maintaining a distinction between being intimate and being dependent is a continuing task. Being close to a woman and taking care of her are two things that sometimes seem to become confused.

Most women involved in the survey said they often tried to hide their stresses from their husbands, fathers, or boyfriends. They felt that men acted overwhelmed, resentful, or defensive when confronted with female stress. Most claimed that what they really needed was to be held and heard, not "helped." Try taking their advice literally. If a woman in your life is stressed, be an active *listener* when she talks. Don't take over or pull back. Try to understand things from her point of view, since her stress is often very different from yours. Do it not only for her sake, but for your own; or you will find that the tension level rises as your stresses and hers compound each other.

7 ON THE JOB: THE STRESSES OF STRIVING

IT'S A BOY! THE DOCTOR ANNOUNCED YOUR BIRTH, AND TRAINING FOR achievement, and all the stress that brings, began. In fact, training for this type of male stress may have begun *before* your birth, with the expectations of your parents.

- In 110 cultures studied by H. Barry, M. Bacon, and I. L. Child, 87 percent of people surveyed expected males to grow up to be more achieving than females, and 85 percent expected males to be more self-reliant as well.

- J. Meyer and B. Soblieszek found that when men were shown videotapes of a seventeen-month-old child and told that they were looking at a girl, they characterized the baby as passive, cuddly, and delicate. When they were told that they were looking at a boy, however, they more often described the baby as active, alert, and aggressive.

- D. Aberle and K. Naegle interviewed fathers about their expectations for their daughters and their sons. There were no surprises: they expected their daughters to be fragile, pretty, and sweet; they expected their sons to be assertive and athletic.

- J. Rubin, F. Provenzano, and Z. Luria suggest that fathers actually perceive their babies to be just what they expect. Fathers looking at their daughters saw them as more awkward, less attentive, softer, finer-featured, and less strong than did fathers looking at their sons. Conversely, fathers looking at their sons saw them as better coordinated, more alert, tougher, larger-featured, firmer, and harder than fathers looking at their daughters. How do these perceptions stack up to the reality? The birth weights, lengths, and reflex times for *all* the babies, girls and boys, were the same in this study!

EARLY ASSERTIVENESS TRAINING

Expectations turn into self-fulfilling prophecies, as parents and other adults begin to treat boys in a way that is consistent with their perceptions and expectations. Parents are less protective of their sons than of their daughters, implicitly teaching their sons that they had better be independent and self-reliant. They compliment their sons on strength and size rather than on looks and manners. Teachers and parents tolerate more aggressiveness from boys than from girls and fathers permit more boasting, assertiveness, and competition in their sons.

Boys are bounced, pounced, roughed up, and tumbled down. They are taught to "take it." They are told: "Put up or shut up." "Talk is cheap." "Fight your own battles." "Get out there and win." "Make us proud of you."

From Little League to the big leagues is a short jump. The message is the same: "Don't let the team down. We're counting on you." The more prominent the player, the more pressure to perform. At first, you perform for your parents. Later, for your peers. Finally, for yourself. But that does not diminish performance pressure. In fact, living up to your own demands is likely to be the most stressful experience of all!

At work, the striving man has not only internalized early expectations for achievement, assertiveness, and reward, but he has usually added messages of his own. He chooses goals and grades himself continually. Whether it's salary, title, office size or location, number of subordinates, degrees, or awards, they are merely symbols of his quest. The winning is more important than the win itself, and every success means a new, higher goal must be set. As one sports medicine physician describes the dilemma: "No man ever wants less than he has become used to, although that is usually more than he needs."

Early assertiveness training is not the legacy of white-collar, button-down-collar, or tab-collar families only, nor are the effects of the stress of striving restricted to executive jobs. Young urban professionals, mature executives, auto mechanics, and crane operators may be equally driven by performance concerns and competitive feelings. Different types of occupational positions, however, do mean different types of stress scenarios. For the decision-maker, responsibility comes with power. For the team worker or employee, lack of responsibility for decisions may also mean a loss of control over working pace, or conditions, or terms. Either scenario can be frustrating, even more so if the man is a Type A or even a Type A+ personality! Let's examine each scenario in turn.

THE RESPONSIBILITY FACTOR

Taking control over decision-making cannot be avoided if you want to be successful in any job or profession—even more so if you are in business for yourself. It is, in fact, a sign of striving for success. It reflects goal-oriented thinking and the self-reliant behavior taught to boys at their parents' knees. It is a healthy extension of the early need to explore, crawl, walk, and run. It is a positive way of gaining self-esteem and others' esteem. It is even a natural way of trying to reduce stress. After all, the more we take control of life decisions, the more predictable life becomes, and the fewer unexpected fight, flight, or fright experiences are thrust upon us.

Since our stress seems to decrease as our sense of control increases, having choices and making decisions should lead to fewer stressful experiences and symptoms. Why, then, is the person in charge—the boss, small business man, or executive—generally highly stressed? The answer is the "responsibility factor."

The stress of constant rising expectations is matched by constant rising responsibilities at work. Supervisors, union workshop leaders, and managers are still team players, but they are now responsible for many or all of the plays. They may be credited with wins, but the losses are theirs also. With added control over planning comes the added responsibility for strategy decisions. This is the key to what is often called "executive stress," even though it is certainly not exclusive to executives! Here are the specific stresses that go hand-in-hand with increased responsibility:

1. *The stress of anticipation.* The consequences of each decision grow with the magnitude of each decision. Therefore, higher-level managers must try to cope with and consider more possible hitches and glitches than those on lower levels. Some have trouble falling asleep worrying about tomorrow's fallout from today's decisions. Some wake up early just to get a head start anticipating possible problems for the new day.

2. *The stress of visibility.* The more important or far-reaching the decision, the more questions about the decision-maker are usually asked and answered. It is difficult to remain private if the decisions you must handle have consequences for co-workers, subordinates, or superiors. If you are in politics, the consequences of your actions are particularly public. If you are in business for yourself, you may be responsible for employees, patients, or clients. When you are working

for your father and make a poor decision, you may be bawled out; if you are working for yourself and make a bad decision, you may have to declare bankruptcy.

3. *The stress of success.* Every success sets new standards for your performance, not only in the eyes of others, but in your eyes as well. With successes come promotions, with promotions come new tasks and responsibilities. As quotas go up, so does stress.

4. *The stress of failure.* Not every decision achieves its intended effect. At lower levels of the hierarchy, a less-than-successful decision-maker might be given a chance to learn from his mistake. At higher levels, the policy is more likely to be identifying responsibility for unsuccessful decisions and eliminating the potential for costly mistakes by eliminating the decision-maker.

Many of the men I interviewed who work for large companies described an "up or out" policy. That is, many companies have fewer and fewer positions at each level of upper management, so they must promote or fire middle-level employees as new trainees join the ranks. "Look around you," employees are told. "One of the two people sitting next to you will probably not be here next year."

Such a policy certainly accentuates the stresses of anticipation, visibility, success, and failure—all the ingredients of "executive stress." But executive stress is not only a result of corporate policy or company structure. Men often bring their own stresses to the office along with their attaché cases and newspapers.

MOVING UP, BURNING OUT

In *The Corporate Steeplechase,* Srully Blotnick outlines four of the "inner" stresses that those on the management level struggle with. After interviewing five thousand business people over a period of twenty-five years, he found that men bring different worries to their work at different ages.

- In his twenties, the entry-level businessman worries about living up to his own image of success. The confident claims and name-dropping that were part of his initial interview now haunt him. Can he really do the job? Can he fill his own shoes? Will he feel like an imposter? Will he look like a fraud? The young business-woman often faces the work world with too few role models to guide her; the young businessman often feels that he has too many to live up to.

- In his thirties, he worries about standing out and being noticed while functioning as a team player. If he tries to go it alone, he is likely to be sabotaged by co-workers or even fired for functioning too autonomously. If he melds into the crowd, moving up becomes unlikely.

- In his forties, the "dangerous decade," the executive experiences a double stress-threat. The younger genera-tion may be pushing their way up from beneath him, and the older generation may be blocking his advance-ment from above. "Burnout" may really represent being *burned up* about being stuck or unsuccessful!

- In his fifties and beyond, an executive should be enjoy-ing his position of elder statesman, his corporate know-how, and his political savvy. Many become mentors and receive major promotions. But more become stressed by a sense of loss of control over a difficult national econo-my or their own future in their jobs. Retirement may be mandatory and protégés may become antagonists. In fact, 40 percent of protégés get fired by their own men-tors, according to Dr. Blotnick.

If you are an executive, manager, self-employed professional, or business owner you may suspect that "executive stress" does not end here. If you deal with clients, then you must worry about their moods as well as your own. Criteria for success may hinge on their opinions, and your reputation may be only as good as your last success. If contracts or clients go elsewhere, your job may be lost with their revenue.

If your product is a creative concept, as with architects, designers, decorators, and artists, your success/failure may ride on timing, fads, publicity, or endorsement. You must use judgment but avoid being judgmental, or you may "freeze" creatively. You must be original, but avoid being seen as too bizarre to be commercial. You must continue to grow and change, but not lose the style that is identifiably yours.

Among the self-employed, farmers may be the most stressed. "There is a feeling of being out of control," says Richard Murdocco of the State University of New York at Stony Brook in a *New York Times* article. Farmers have no control over the weather or prices of their products. Add to these stressors seven-day workweeks, few vacations, if any, and constant financial worries, and you have a whole population at high risk for stress-related illness.

In a highly competitive business, "you must worry not only about moving up, but staying in," according to psychologist Diana Powell. High job insecurity is always a condition for high stress. In the early 1980s, behavioral consultant Ron Edelson sampled one thousand accountants, lawyers, and ad-agency professionals and, as expected, found a higher percentage of stress-related cardiovascular, respiratory, digestive, and mental illnesses among the group with the least job security—advertising agency professionals. And Melvin Glasser, in a 1984 essay, noted that worrying about their employment termination led to a 700 percent increase in heart attacks and stress illnesses among ground controllers for the Apollo space project toward the end of that project in 1969.

Job insecurity, however, has become almost everyone's problem in the 1990s due to economic downturns and corporate "downsizing." Herbert Nieberg, a clinical psychologist and employee assistance professional in Westchester County, New York, says that job stress, which began rising in the 1980s, has become epidemic in the 1990s. What has changed in the 1990s is the more pervasive feeling of insecurity and anxiety. Not only are the people who lost their jobs under a great deal of stress, so are the "survivors"—the ones who have been spared in the latest round of layoffs, for example. These survivors may very well develop stress-related conditions, too, because they're constantly worrying about whether they will be next to go and because they're working twice as hard to fill the void left by their departed co-workers. According to Dr. Nieberg, the older male managers have the most difficulty with job loss and feelings of worthlessness that come with it and their family members—the wife and children—may catch the stress if the man does not get help.

And last, but not least, if you are in the sales arena, or selling your personality to the public, as performers and politicians do, you recognize stress that Gail Matthews, a psychologist at Dominican College in San Rafael, California, calls the "imposter phenomenon"—a fear of being "found out." She surveyed lawyers, judges, physicians, priests, police, writers, and scientists. The most famous felt the most of this kind of stress since their work could not be measured by objective standards. "What would happen," they worried, "if I stopped working so hard? Would everyone see that I am not gifted, but only more driven?" So they don't stop.

SUCCESS DISTRESS

If you are very successful you may have yet one more executive stress to deal with: success distress. Most of us would say that we wouldn't mind dealing with the stress of success, but many researchers have found that the idea of success distress is more amusing than the reality.

Ralph thought twice and then three times before he joined his brother in a real-estate venture. Together they bought an old brownstone on Manhattan's West Side and began to renovate it. Ralph was an accountant, not an entrepreneur, and he felt uncomfortable investing speculatively. But the venture was profitable, and Ralph next joined his brother in an ice cream franchise located directly across the street from New York's busiest movie theater complex. Soon Ralph's investments had made him wealthy and his accounting practice was secondary in terms of his income, though not his time. The practice he had worked so hard to develop would have put him into the middle class; his business ventures made him rich. He did not feel lucky—he felt anxious and depressed, and he did not know why.

The anxiety and depression Ralph was feeling after his financial success tell us that he did not feel entitled to it. He had always expected to work very hard for awards and rewards. Multiplying his money his brother's way felt too easy. And "easy come" sometimes means "easy go." He had no sense of control with regard to his investments. Right moves on his brother's part meant riches; would wrong moves lead to rags? A high sense of luck, low sense of control, and a questionable sense of entitlement are the hallmarks of success distress.

Guilt plays a role here, too. Many successful people compare themselves to those less fortunate and feel guilty. They wait superstitiously for some disaster so that "cosmic equity" will be restored. The more successful they are, the greater the disaster they expect. Madeline Hirschfeld, a New York psychologist, notes that these people can create the very disasters they expect. Their guilt leads to self-deprecating and self-defeating statements. After a while, they and others start to believe!

Feeling good can have you feeling bad for yet another reason. We are all creatures of habit, and some of us are used to feeling bad. *The New York Times* quotes Henry Sedgwick, an investment banker, as saying that feeling good can be so unfamiliar that people want to go back to something they are used to dealing with. The joy of achievement is, therefore, eclipsed by the distress of success. It took Sedgwick four years to resume investing after his first big success!

WHEN IT'S ONLY A JOB:
THE LOW-CONTROL FACTOR

Some men find it hard to sympathize with success distress. They laugh and say, "I only wish I had *that* problem. I'm too busy taking orders to worry about the stresses of *giving* orders or dealing with success!"

What about those who enter the work force not as executive trainees or professionals, but as workers, those who take orders rather than give them? What happens to the expectations for achievement that they have been building up? What happens to those stress patterns we have been describing?

- "I'm a short-order cook. That's my trade. That's all that I know. I've been doing it for thirty, thirty-five years. How many ways can you make a scrambled egg?"

- "I'm a traffic cop. When I started out I thought it was a big deal. And then the girls were small—I have three daughters. They came around and watched me sometimes. They thought I was great. I liked that. I thought I was pretty good, too. But now I feel like it's just a job—a job with a uniform. Anyone can do it."

- "I'm a doorman. I've been at this place a couple of years. It's okay; nothing special. The time I like is early in the morning, six o'clock or so. It's quiet and not too hot. You can talk to somebody like a human being. Later there's always something, even when you're not that busy. At night you're just tired. Not satisfied."

- "I'm a salesman. This place I'm working at might lose its lease. Nobody knows yet. What the owner has in mind— I have no idea. He doesn't tell me anything. How can I plan my life?"

Achievement, self-reliance, and assertiveness are every bit as important to the stress dynamics of the nonexecutive's day as they are to the executive's. Loss of control, loss of esteem, and loss of position trigger the fight and flight response for both, but the battlegrounds for the fight and the options for the flight are very different. The battleground for nonexecutives is filled with *workplace routines, workplace conditions,* and *workplace risks,* which multiply their stress experiences and undermine their stress-coping patience. What I am saying is that it is potentially *more* stressful to be a nonexecutive achieving personality than it is to be an executive achiever.

WORKPLACE ROUTINES

Repeated routines sound easy and relaxing, and this may be true when they are recreational routines. It's definitely *not* true, however, when they are required occupational routines. In fact, a study by Robert Caplan and associates found that workers on machine-paced assembly lines have the highest stress and strain of any of twenty-three occupations they studied. These were workers who reported "the most boredom and the greatest dissatisfaction with the workload." Their jobs mean low participation, low complexity of work, and low utilization of abilities. In other words, the assembly line leaves no room for achievement, self-reliance, or assertiveness. The short-order cook makes breakfast thousands of times a year. The policeman faces the same gridlock every day at four o'clock. The doorman opens the same door again and again.

Routine jobs produce specialists, but they are self-limiting ("How many ways can you make a scrambled egg?") Routine jobs produce autonomy, but they are isolating (nobody told the salesman anything about losing the lease). Routine jobs produce familiarity, but they are frustrating ("At night you're just tired. Not satisfied").

Shift work is a routine that has its own special kinds of stress. Sometimes the stress results from mismatches—forcing "night" people to work during the day and "day" people to work during the night. Even if there are no mismatches, shift work *still* requires seventy-two hours for the body to readjust itself. According to Leon J. Warshaw, executive director of the New York

Business Group on Health, the most stressful form of shift work is the rotating type, in which workers switch every few weeks or so. In fact, in the two or three days after shift changes, the accident rate goes up and productivity goes down—until the body adjusts to the new routine. Many specialists in sleep disorders have blamed a number of plane crashes and even the nuclear accident at Three-Mile Island on sleep deprivation caused by such shift work changes.

WORKPLACE CONDITIONS

Men at managerial, professional, and executive as well as non-executive levels sometimes feel that their jobs leave no room for "masculine" qualities, no room to exercise control. But executives can at least suffer the resultant stress in air-conditioned offices, where the noises are reduced, the dust is filtered out, the lights are bright, and the secretaries talk softly. For most workingmen, the actual working conditions are not a refuge from stress, they're an additional source of it.

Among the major problems are noise, heat, dust, odors, and poor lighting. In fact, it's been estimated by Melvin Glasser that *40 percent* of U.S. workers are exposed to injurious noise levels, greater than seventy decibels—the sound of a light vacuum cleaner fifteen feet away. Remember the research study referred to in Chapter 3 which found that when the noise level is high in the workplace, men respond with higher levels of tension, blood pressure, and heart rate? And Harold Visotsky cites the case of computer keypunch operators and word processors—in his words, "one of the largest stress groups because so much eyestrain occurs." Dr. Visotsky found that if these workers were given a fifteen-minute break every hour, their productivity rose by 25 percent!

Perhaps the most dramatic, and tragic, example of stress in the workplace is the virtual epidemic of murders and suicides involving postal workers. In the last decade, thirty-four people were killed and twenty were wounded by postal workers who took revenge for the loss of a job or for a reprimand by a supervisor. Many postal employees and experts in workplace violence blame the Postal Services' factory-like conditions and a high-pressured, hostile, and authoritarian atmosphere for the violence. The postal workers allege that sorting letters on machines at the rate of one per second, lifting and throwing countless packages per day, and working at a pace mandated by management all set the stage for high rates of injury as well.

WORKPLACE RISKS

Heat, noise, odors, and poor lighting can certainly create stress, but for some, workplace conditions are actual hazards to health, risks to lives. Obvious examples are building construction projects, bridge-painting jobs, and demolition work—jobs in which the risk of injury or death is ever-present and inescapable. Other working risks are more subtle: for example, exposure to substances such as asbestos and fiber dust, and certain exhaust gases, chemical products, and similar substances known or suspected to be agents of cancer or other serious illnesses.

These conditions pose two problems. One is the actual risk to health. The other is the fact that as these hazards become known, the stress of the workers increases—and the known hazards become publicized in the work force very quickly.

This kind of stress can be uniquely hard to handle, because it strikes at the heart of the need for control. On the one hand, the worker can leave the job and give up control of his career, his livelihood, and his sense of worth. On the other hand, he can stay on the job and give up control over his body, knowing that his body is being attacked eight hours a day, five days a week, and *there's nothing he can do about it.*

THE COMPANY POLICY BLUES

Apart from job routines and working conditions, what the company as a whole does clearly affects all its employees. But with their smaller sense of participation and power, it doesn't make much difference to low-level employees whether the company's actions are a short-term response to market conditions or the result of long-established policies.

As far as the worker is directly concerned, what the company can do is fire him, retire him, move him, change his job, or let him stew in rumors without denying or confirming them. They're all potent sources of stress. Leon Warshaw compiled a group of nineteen job-related "stressors." At the top of the list is loss of job *security*. This is more serious, says Dr. Warshaw, than loss of the job itself (just as unpredictable consequences are often harder to take than known negative consequences). In other words, rumors of layoffs and firings can be as stressful or more stressful than actually being laid off. Consider these other items on Dr. Warshaw's list of workplace stressors:

- loss of job through forced retirement
- job change through relocation
- job change through promotion
- changes within the job through shift-work changes
- work overload without recourse
- work unload, leading to boredom or less income
- unforeseen deadlines
- inappropriate work hours
- unhealthy or unpleasant work conditions
- too much job competition
- too little cooperation
- inadequate information supply to workers
- inadequate routes for input into company decisions
- ambiguous or conflicting job duties
- too little recognition of achievement
- too few promotion opportunities
- inadequate financial return
- no incentives or special privileges

These "stressors" have been studied and identified in factories and in fieldwork, in bureaucracies and in department stores. Most men who responded to the Male Stress Survey mentioned at least one. Many mentioned more than one. And in a study conducted by Joseph N. Ruocco, it was found that most of these same stressors plague men throughout the Western World.

NONEXECUTIVE BURNOUT

We read much about executive burnout, and here we are discussing nonexecutive burnout. What does the term "burnout" really mean? According to Fred Charatran of the Long Island Jewish-Hillside Medical Center, burnout is a "kind of secret, internal, psychological flight" from your work. It's a disengagement from work, removing all feelings of importance and interest from it.

Internally, burnout is a psychological symptom of depression; on the job, it usually results in lower efficiency, lower morale, and higher job turnover rates, with the following results:

Accidents and Illness
According to Edward J. Cleary, President of the New York State A.F.L.-C.I.O., one U.S. worker dies every hour of every day, every year—10,000 per year overall. Six million are injured on the job each year and 60,000 are permanently disabled. Melvin Glasser, in his 1984 essay "Labor Looks at Work Stress," is sure that a large part of these injuries and deaths is the result of stress.

The moral is clear: As job stresses increase, your chances of getting hurt or sick on the job increase also. The solution is first to recognize these stressful work situations and assume that if at least one of them applies to you, you're under stress. Then do your best to control it, cancel it, or work it off, following the stress management techniques given in Chapter 9.

Job Performance
The three classic effects of job stress are absenteeism, accidents, and alcoholism. We've talked about accidents and, in Chapter 3, alcoholism, and of course these also contribute to absenteeism. So do burnout and burnout-related states—feeling that the job is not worth your energy, or that you have no energy to give it.

There's another way of responding to on-the-job stress, however, that's exactly the opposite. It's an attempt to gain a sense of job control by working harder, longer, and with greater determination.

Sherman A. James and associates at the University of North Carolina School of Public Health, examined the relationship between education level, diastolic blood pressure level, and scores on a performance motivation scale among 132 males. Those subjects who scored highest on this scale and low on education level also had significantly higher diastolic blood pressure than their less driven co-workers. Thus, those with this pattern, unrelieved by stress-coping approaches that might be learned at higher education levels, develop a system of internal, self-generated stresses to help them cope with external, job- or life-generated stresses. But as far as the body is concerned, stress is stress and high blood pressure is high blood pressure, and they're both bad for you.

NONSTRESS STRATEGIES FOR WORKPLACE STRESSORS

When it comes to job or work stress control, there are three areas to concentrate on: your own reactions, your support network, and your employer.

Personal Stress Control

Stress control by you, the individual, must begin with an awareness of *when* you are under stress. Besides your own internal awareness, the early warning signals in Chapter 4 are helpful. Then practice the stress reduction techniques described in Chapter 9, to keep from being harmed by stressful situations you can't do anything about; and take action against those stressors you *can* change. Taking control and making choices will help lower your stress levels.

Help from the Family

Family members who want to help a man under stress have to

take the same first step as the individual himself: recognize when stress is involved. Then:

1. Suggest the stress control measures we've discussed here, or suggest that he read the appropriate chapters in this book himself.

2. Encourage his participation in stress burnoff techniques—both physical activity and emotional outlets. And don't forget the healing properties of laughter. Look for opportunities to laugh together.

3. Encourage a rest period after work stress. For many men (and women) twenty minutes *alone* when they first come home from work is as effective as a cocktail. At least, when everyone comes home from work, keep new problems away from discussion for a reasonable period of time.

4. Above all, encourage him to talk. This is not always easy to do, because many men resist talking over their problems—*especially* with their families. They want to retain their Superman image. These men may talk to their doctors, however. So, if the man in your family is showing signs of stress, he's probably also showing some physical reason for visiting a doctor, and a little advance planning on your part with the doctor might be very helpful in directing him toward stress management.

Help from the Employer

Just as the first goal of the workingman and his family is to recognize stress when it occurs, the first goal of the employer is to recognize that stress in an employee is bad for the company. Accidents and absenteeism mean less production, longer delays, and lower quality, and they're all directly related to employee stress.

Just as it's important for the worker and his family to know what stress consists of before they can fight it, it's important for employers to know what *nonstress* is before they can create it. Here, Melvin Glasser offers some suggestions. In a survey of automobile workers, the five items of greatest importance in their work were:

- to belong
- to receive recognition
- to know what goes on
- to be able to talk to their bosses
- to be proud of their jobs

If your employer seems unaware of this information, as well as other stressors affecting your productivity, try suggesting one or more of the following:

1. A breakfast meeting once a week, or once a month, with a group of workers or a few representatives of different groups. Ideas can then be exchanged in a relaxed atmosphere.

2. A joint employee-employer venture to provide counseling opportunities for stressed employees. An on-site psychologist, a community counseling center, or a group leader can offer lunch-hour sessions and referral services for physical and psychological problems.

3. An exercise program, meditation class, and/or rest area. Co-workers are often skilled enough in at least one of these areas to provide the leadership for the programs as long as your employer will designate the facility.

4. An employee-conducted survey of positive productivity-enhancing suggestions. Passing such a survey on to your employer indicates your interest in the company while it increases your sense of belonging, communication with management, recognition, and identification with company success.

ARE YOU A TYPE A?

Do you have to be an executive to call yourself a Type A man? *NO!* Although high-achieving men frequently show many of the characteristics that Meyer Friedman and Ray Rosenman correlated with stress-related heart disease in their research for *Type A Behavior and Your Heart*, most men show at least one of the characteristics. Showing many Type A behaviors makes you Super Type A's—what I call a Type A+ personality. But showing even *one* makes you a Type A man.

My Type A patients generally describe themselves in the following ways. How many describe you, too? Remember, even one "yes" is enough to make you a Type A:

I am never satisfied with my achievements.

I am impatient with myself.

I am impatient with others (but try to hide it).

I overschedule myself to the point that one traffic jam throws my whole day off.

I am a stimulus junky; I prefer too much to do to too little to do.

I feel I work better under pressure, so I often let projects pile up until I am under the gun.

I am openly competitive at sports, but a closet competitor at work. That is, I secretly assess others' progress and then expect even more of myself.

I expect so very much of myself that I cannot tolerate any further demands or criticism.

I experience telephone tension. Every ringing telephone represents a new problem for me to solve.

I hate to wait!

I have a quick temper, which I try to hide (and pay the price in migraines, high blood pressure, or angina).

I am not sure I am really lovable, so work becomes my world.

I am not sure that I can control my family's feelings, so work becomes my world.

I have "status insecurity," so work becomes my world.

In therapy, these men often discover that they felt unaccepted as children—unseen, unloved, or both. Their current life becomes a continual series of "do-overs." Through work they try to make their mark: be seen, be admired, earn love through power, prestige, and money. All these attempts, of course, do not solve the original problem, so each success does not yet satisfy. The more accurate solution involves accepting parents as people who had shortcomings. If they, indeed, neglected their child or gave only conditional love, it was not because the child had a problem or was unlovable. In other words, it was not the child's fault. The early situation cannot be corrected and, instead, must be *left behind.* The Type A+ man must *certainly* move on, learn to parent himself.

HOW TO BE A "B"

Once a Type A, always a Type A? Probably, but you can learn some survival techniques from Type B, or low-stress, personalities. A Type B is at lower risk for male stress symptoms because:

- He is not as stressed by setbacks or failures, since his expectations for himself and for life are more realistic than optimistic.

- He is not as obsessed by past glories or future fantasies, since he accepts who he is today, rather than focusing on who he was yesterday or who he should be tomorrow.

- He is not as impatient or interfering when he delegates responsibility, since he is less competitive than a Type A and less likely to personalize others' behaviors.

- He is not as perfectionistic, since he has a greater sense of security, and is not as approval-seeking, since he has a greater sense of self-esteem.

- He doesn't overschedule himself as often, since he is more likely to do what he *can* do than to try to do what he thinks he *should* do.

- He is not as self-conscious about playing, dancing, chancing something new, or laughing out loud, since he is not monitoring his behavior for "appearances."

- He is not as apt to have trouble giving and receiving affection and compliments, since he has less free-floating hostility.

The Type B doesn't tap his foot compulsively, or finish sentences for others. The Type B doesn't clench his jaw in jealousy, or critically reevaluate himself when others show off their successes. The Type B doesn't feel his heart race when the traffic doesn't.

Although the goals of a Type B man are usually more realistic and less demanding than those of a Type A, Type B behavior is not incompatible with hard work and achievement. What is missing from the Type B profile is not motivation, but time urgency, hostility, and insecurity. This leaves energy for reading, writing, musing, and amusing. This leaves the Type B more free time each day, and probably also means he will have more days!

Of course, Type A's and Type B's are merely profiles on paper; no one is a perfect Type A or B. The more the Type B profile fits, however, the lower the risk for cardiovascular trouble, according to most research. How does one acquire Type B behavior?

I have often told my clients and my patients that Type B behavior is a gift. It can be given to you by your parents when you are growing up, or you can *give it to yourself as a present now*! Parents who give their children unconditional acceptance and love give them the gift of Type B behavior, because the child feels that his talents as well as his shortcomings are recognized. He does not have to be perfect to be a person worth loving. Fathers who can best make their sons feel this way are usually Type B fathers themselves. More than Type A fathers, they have the time and patience to notice their sons' small victories, sympathize with their small disappointments, and listen to their small voices. Their sons, in turn, are learning how to treat others with love and patience, and how to treat themselves the same way.

If this was not your parental legacy, today is the day to begin parenting yourself—the Type B way! It took years of practice for you to perfect your Type A behavior, so don't expect to be a B overnight. But don't think your behavior can't be changed, either. Here is how you begin:

Make Your Own Physical and Mental Health a Priority
Don't use yourself as cheap labor. Don't abuse yourself by depriving yourself of your emotional needs. Don't practice mental cruelty toward yourself by expecting that you can carry on at all costs—the cost is often too steep. If you begin to take care of yourself as conscientiously as you like to be taken of, much of your Type A behavior will begin to change.

Get to Know Yourself as You Are
We all know who we think we *should* be, and some of us know who we would *like* to be; few of us know who we actually *are*. Sit down today and start a self-description list. Add only one item to the list each day. Live that entire day with a heightened awareness of the aspect of yourself that you have added to the list. If, for example, the first item is "I am competitive," spend a day noticing what situations trigger your competitive reactions, how useful or realistic these reactions are, and how frequently you react this way. Gathering this information gives you a starting point for modification. You may want to avoid some triggering situations, or try out other reactions instead. Criticizing yourself and berating your competitiveness will not lead to self-esteem or positive change; self-knowledge can lead to both.

Re-Examine Your Sense of Time Urgency
Type A personalities typically attribute much of whatever success they have achieved to their pattern of making every moment count. They feel that they accomplish double by doing two things at once, or by doing two things in the time needed for just the first project. In fact, according to Meyer Friedman and Diane Ulmer, they accomplish no more than Type B per-

sonalities accomplish. This is because the Type A "hurry sickness" produces impatience, irritation, aggravation, and anger as its side effects. Remember the British study mentioned in Chapter 3? Type A's working against a deadline had blood pressure readings that were twice as high as those who worked at their own pace. Ironically, the self-paced group completed the task in the same amount of time as those who hurried to meet the deadline! In this case, too, impatience, irritation, aggravation, and anger complicated the task at hand. These four emotions interfere with efficiency and leave Type A's falling further and further behind their own quota levels. The alternative? In their book *Treating Type A Behavior and Your Heart*, Friedman and Ulmer suggest that Type A personalities re-examine their achievements in order to identify the real reasons for their success:

- creativity
- decision-making ability
- organization
- leadership ability
- broad perspectives
- determination

Once a Type A has identified the real reason or reasons for his success, he can begin to dare to give up his constant sense of time urgency.

Give Yourself Permission to Play

Instead of sending your children into another room to play after your hard day, *join them*. This will give you a Type B break from work, a chance to capture a fleeting moment in your children's rapid sprint from infancy to teens, and, I trust, some fun. Instead of steaming when your roommate puts up his feet and opens the newspaper to try the crossword puzzle, join him. You don't feel angry if you don't feel deprived. Instead of just reading restaurant notices, movie reviews, and theater previews, call some friends and join them there. Don't wait until the world gives you permission to take a break—by then you probably won't have the energy for fun. Relaxation and recuperation are *not* synonymous!

Shift Your Focus from Self-Involved to Self-Centered

Type A behavior is usually very self-involved behavior. This means constant spectatoring, checking out your progress or success by trying to see yourself in other people's eyes. Instead of trying to read other people's minds, a Type A can profit more from reading his own. Look at others and at yourself through your *own* eyes. This is what I mean by being self-centered. Type B personalities take the long view and realize that only the future will prove that a current decision or action was a good idea. Type B's usually see their best as good enough; Type A's rarely do.

Practice, Practice

Most psychotherapists will tell you that insight alone will not change long-standing habitual behavior. Learning a new behavior, like learning a new skill or sport, necessitates practice. In his study of 1,012 postinfarction (post-heart attack) subjects, Meyer Friedman found that those who practiced various Type B behavior drills for three years had 372 percent fewer recurrences of heart attacks than did subjects who similarly watched their diet and exercised, but who did not modify their Type A behavior. What exciting statistics!

Dr. Friedman, now in his eighties, is involved in a ten-year study on the possible preventive effects of behavioral counseling. Unlike his previous study, which involved only heart attack patients, the current study will look at the incidence of both coronary artery disease and cancer among more than 3,000 *healthy* Type A's in San Francisco and Connecticut. The results of this study should show how effective behavioral changes are in preventing disease. Here are some of the drills Dr. Friedman uses to modify behavior:

1. Do only one thing at a time. Do not engage in poly-

phasic (more than one thing at a time) activity. When you read, eat, or speak on the telephone, concentrate on that one activity only.

2. Catch yourself when you use quantity rather than quality adjectives in your thoughts or speech. Try to describe the beauty of an object or location without referring to its dollar value.

3. Read books that are purely recreational for you, not occupationally or professionally relevant. Concentrate on the prose as well as the content; look up new words in the dictionary as you encounter them.

4. Walk, eat, and talk more slowly. Drive in the slow lane to avoid pressing the gas pedal with every urgent thought and to achieve a steady, moderate pace as a driving habit.

5. Select times to leave your watch at home. How often did you find yourself looking at your wrist that day?

6. Record your half of a business telephone conversation, or record a dinner conversation with your wife, and play it back to yourself. Note whether or not you are speaking rapidly, asking questions, and listening to answers. Do you try to speed up your conversation by supplying the endings of sentences for your partner? If you recognize a Type A speech pattern, re-record as you practice your listening and Type B conversation skills.

7. Get on the *longest* toll line to practice waiting without agitation. Discover how you can make the time pass pleasantly. Speculate about the lives of those around you. Review pleasant memories. Plan a future trip or project.

8. Check your face in a mirror at least twice a day for signs of annoyance, tension, or fatigue. Get to know these expressions so that you can feel them on your face without looking in the mirror.

9. Practice smiling and laughing. Do this by deliberately thinking of a delightful memory or funny incident. Don't wait for smiles and laughter to come to you— make them happen.

10. Make your implicit spiritual point of view explicit. Review and reappraise your ideas about birth, life, maturity, and even death, whether they are religious, philosophical, or pragmatic in origin. As I advise my patients, students, and readers:

   Turn your palm up and look at your lifeline (the line that starts between the thumb and first finger and curves around the base of the thumb to the wrist). It has a beginning, a middle, and an end. It does not go on forever. Be reminded whenever you look at your hand that life, too, does not go on forever. The time to modify your behavior is now.

8 MARRIAGE, MID-LIFE, AND MYTHS OF AGING

MEN ARE RAISED TO TAKE CHARGE,
> but they cannot all be their own bosses.

Men are raised to be primary providers,
> but they find they are now living during inflation and recession.

Men are raised to focus on achievement,
> but success is usually a momentary experience.

Men are raised to stand on their own,
> but they need support systems.

Men are raised to express "strong" emotions,
> but they often feel "weak" ones like fear and sadness, too.

Men are raised to be team players,
> but it's often "Every man for himself."

Men are raised to be Daddy's Big Boy,
> but expected to remain Mommy's Little Man.

Men are raised to be independent,
> but urged to bond and nest.

Men are raised to follow their dreams,
> but required to be realistic about security.

Men must deal every day with mixed messages about the meaning of being male. They must try to reconcile the lone-wolf image with the one-of-the-guys image; the handyman image with the helpless-at-home image; the family-man image with the do-your-own-thing image; the stiff-upper-lip image with the let-it-all-hang-out image; the all-male image with the sensitive-man image; and the laid-back image with the star image.

And it's not just the media that is sending these mixed messages. Men have their own expectations for themselves based on their early models, reinforcement, and interactions—and too often these expectations do not match the actual man. Men have their own expectations based on the roles they occupy: son, husband, father, professional, friend—and too often these role expectations conflict. Men have their own expectations based on who they would like to be—and too often these expectations are inconsistent with the men they are becoming.

There are, then, three levels of frustrating confusion. First, society's expectations for men are often in conflict. Second, the individual's expectations for himself are often in conflict with society's expectations. And third, a man's many expectations for himself may be in conflict with each other.

It is no wonder that study after study measures high levels of free-floating hostility among adult men. They claim they are trying to be logical and emotional at the same time; successfully competitive, but appropriately cooperative; stable, but spontaneous; protective, but liberated. The interviews I conducted for the Male Stress Survey revealed hopes of total success but terror of total failure; striving for maturity but mourning over lost youth. Such polarity would make anyone's head spin. Such ambivalence would make anyone upset. Such contradictions would make anyone confused. Add the fear of failure, performance anxiety, spectatoring, and competitive compulsions, which were discussed in earlier chapters, and you have the makings of the Male Stress Syndrome. Manhood requires making decisions, or having decisions thrust on you, that will shape the rest of your life. Marriage: now, later, never? Career: for now, until later, forever? Retirement: early, late, forced? Manhood requires that facts and fallacies about divorce, fatherhood, and sexual functioning be sorted out and perhaps confronted.

STRESS AND STRUGGLES WITH ANGER

More than 80 percent of the men who took the Male Stress Survey said they had been physically violent at some point during their lives—some while at war, some while in love, some when at play, and some in self-defense. Why is male conflict so common? I suspect it is in part because of the internal conflicts they must live with. Their inner fights become outer fights. They say they have mixed feelings about religion, marriage, monogamy, and the work ethic. Many, in fact, said that they had mixed feelings about "everything"!

Chronic male anger, then, may be due in part to chronic male agitation about conflicting demands and unresolved attitudes. It may also, however, be overdetermined—that is, it may have more than one cause. Male aggression, overt or covert, may also be due to:

1. *A rehearsal effect.* During their younger years, boys fight. They fight for fun, playing war. They fight for their school, playing sports. They fight for their girl-friends, playing around. Now, as adults, they await the "real thing."

2. *A modeling effect.* Men see men fight in the sports are-nas, in films, on television, as police, as firefighters. They have seen violence "work."

3. *A releasing factor.* Many men experience a surge of aggression when they drink alcohol, which is referred to as a releasing factor. Aggression that they can easi-ly inhibit when they are sober becomes disinhibited when they are intoxicated. If their drinking is the result of being aggravated in the first place, the aggres-

sion released is likely to be particularly volatile.

4. *A rechanneling factor.* As unacceptable as aggression may seem to be, many men have learned that dependency needs, fears, some sexual impulses, sadness, and even love are less acceptable. Tension from these other areas may be rechanneled into the expression of anger or aggressiveness. Homophobia, for example, may be explained as a man's fear of his own more "feminine" emotions being rechanneled into a rage reaction to homosexuals.

5. *A reaction result.* Suppressing and repressing reactions to frustration will not succeed forever. The more a man denies his angry impulses, the more indirectly those impulses are likely to be building force. If he is not recognizing his feelings and using up the adrenaline in a constructive way, he is likely to react rather than act on his feelings.

Chronic anger, like all long-term stresses, wears and tears on psychological and physical resources. It leaves little energy for giving out love, little room for taking in love, and little motivation for making love. So it not only increases the Male Stress Syndrome, it also interferes with avenues of male stress reduction!

TIME TENSION

Fred had been married in his early twenties, for less than a year. Now, in his forties, he told women that he had been married for many years so that they would not think him incapable of having a relationship. But he worried about his capacity for mating after so many years alone. For twenty years he had maintained his weight, his racquetball game, and his attractiveness to women. Last year he broke his ankle and was laid up for three weeks, off racquetball for the season, and in no mood to date. He sat home by himself, gained weight, and worried about growing old alone. His buddies were for the fun times, and his dating

was for the young times. If only he were richer, he thought, or still thirty—"I'd be in a better position to choose a wife and still shape my life."

Men report being acutely aware of time on many levels. They
are aware of the passage of time and that with each year they
may be more bald, more gray, and more rotund. They are aware
of time as a measure of career or financial achievement. They
are aware of time moving them toward stress symptoms that
could be debilitating or fatal. They are aware of time moving
them away from the "good old days" and the "good old guys."

Although men, unlike women, can start new families in their
fifties and even sixties, men in their thirties and forties often
feel an urgency if they have not yet had children. Some men say
they don't want to be too old to throw a ball around with their
son when he is ten. Others say that they don't want to be so
much older than the child's mother that they are taken for the
grandfather. Still others feel an urgent need to decide whether
or not they really want children at all.

Men who have not married are stressed by the passage of
time in two important ways. First, they become increasingly
aware that they may themselves be contributing to their single
state. That is, the older man is less likely to say that he has not
yet found the right woman, and more likely to ask himself if he
could deal with her if he did. As clinical psychologist Bruce
Bernstein explains, older men often begin to ask themselves if
they have the capacity to give love, rather than dwelling on
whether or not they have a woman around to give love to.
Second, men who have not married and are approaching their
middle years speak of the fear of being alone. Although most are
not lonely, they worry that they may become ill or incapacitated, no longer able to date, and, finally, isolated. As one man
put it, "The single man lives like a king, but dies like a dog."

PROVIDING AND STRESS

Listen to the stresses created by the pressure to provide:

"I feel in charge of the world. It's too much."

"I try to juggle my family and my job. Instead, I end up feeling juggled."

"What I dread most is poverty. That keeps me going."

"I learned that hard work brings success. I now think hard work brings hard work."

"I feel that I can do better than I am. I don't just mean money-wise. I mean that I'm not using all my skills, and that upsets me."

"I keep comparing myself to my friends to see how I'm doing. Even though I'm doing fine, I can't stop comparing!"

"It's the doctor's bills and payments on my pension that give me nightmares."

"You may laugh, but I'm always worried about holding up the family name."

"Sometimes I wish I'd get sick so that no one would expect me to take care of them anymore."

"Every birthday I reassess my income. Every birthday I get depressed."

"We need two incomes now, and I feel like a failure. My wife's earning a living— so what's *my* claim to fame?"

Interestingly, it is not only men who are aware of the pressures that go with breadwinning. Wives also worry about their husbands' preoccupation with finances and their jobs. Even women who work outside the house tend not to define themselves in terms of their income—but men often do. Although they are every bit as competitive, women fill so many roles that their work worries are diffused by their other worries about children, parents, friends, homes. For men, work worries are always in focus, undiluted and stress-filled.

SOCIAL ISOLATION

"Who do you talk with when you are stressed?" I asked in interviews. "What do you mean?" they replied. "Who do you turn to when you want to talk something out?" I explained. "No one," they usually said. "Why?" Their answers can be summarized as follows:

- Those men who use occupational success as their standard of self-worth cannot share their feelings with other men because they are concerned about comparing and competing with them instead.

- Men who have been taught assertiveness often feel diminished by admitting to stress.

- Men frequently distrust other men who have information about their "weaknesses."

- Talking is seen by some men as "feminine"; action is expected of men.

- Many men report that they are suspicious of the motivation of men who do not "keep their distance."

- Talking to other men is like asking for opinions, some said. They preferred to minimize rather than maximize others' opinions.

- Sadly, many men said they would like to have the kind of friend they could talk to, but felt that they had invested too much in a macho posture to change their style.

Stoicism, outside of the dental chair, is more dysfunctional than desirable. It deprives men of a sense of bonding or belonging, of different points of view, of networking for resources, of escape valves, of sympathy and empathy, of reassurance, and of objective feedback. As extended families, and even intact families, become less available, extended friendship becomes more vital to the management of stress. Whether it's a cause or an effect, social isolation is correlated with depression and even suicide. Nurture your friendships for your own sake as well as others'.

STRESS AND THE FAMILY MAN

Fewer than 5 percent of American men live their lives without marriage at some point, for some period of time. As of 1992, according to the U.S. Bureau of the Census, 65 percent of American men were currently married and 67 percent were heads of households, whether married, divorced, or widowed. Whereas 80 percent of men between the ages of twenty and twenty-four are single, only 18 percent of men between thirty-five and thirty-nine are single. By the time men reach their mid- to late forties, only 7 percent of them are single!

Exposure to some stresses of marriage, then, is almost inevitable for men; exposure to the stresses that go with fathering is probable; and exposure to the acute stresses of divorcing is frequent. Although married men do live longer than never-married men, divorced men, or widowers, it is not because family life is stress-free. The family serves many functions at its best—but it is certainly not always functioning at its best.

FUNCTIONING AND DYSFUNCTIONING MARRIAGES

Why are more than 1,200,000 men signing up for marriage every year? Particularly in an era when live-in relationships are more popular than ever before? Psychologists, psychiatrists, anthropologists, and sociologists agree, for the most part, that the family structure has many positive assets to offer:

1. Marriage offers a continuity that counteracts stress. A married man can predict with some assurance what activities will fill his weekends, what financial needs will arise, what holidays will be celebrated and with whom, and what his sexual life will be like. The less

predictable these areas of life, the more stressful they are. The high death risk of widowers and divorced men, compared to married men the same age, certainly seems to make the same point.

According to the 1994 *Merck Manual of Geriatrics*, in the first week after the death of a spouse, the expected mortality rate for the remaining spouse doubles, and death usually results from a heart attack. In the first three months after the death of a spouse, the mortality rate increases 48 percent in men sixty-five and older. Widowed men who remain unmarried continue to have a higher-than-expected death rate up to ten years after the death of the spouse. This higher mortality rate may be due to the fact that men living alone neglect their nutritional, health care, and psychological needs. In his book *The First Year of Bereavement*, Ira Glick reminds us that many men confide *only* in their wives and are losing their best friend when she dies.

2. Married life provides for the upbringing and financial support of children. The family unit is the source of role models, rewards, punishments, and resources for growing children. The children themselves offer the family a source of pride, fun, vicarious youth, and the preservation of family name and tradition.

3. A husband and wife can give each other an emotional support system and loving network. Friendships may offer this also, but not as intimately and continuously as marriage can. Love from those who have seen you at your worst as well as your best is true love, indeed.

4. Two cannot really live as cheaply as one, but two incomes can double your purchasing power. Many families function best as an economic unit, and couples pool their resources for long-range financial goals in a way that dating men do not or cannot.

5. Marriage can be a forum for communication. Sometimes, in fact, it is the only forum for secret fears, silli-

ness, anger, hurt, or tears, which men hide from the rest
of the world. Ideally, a man can talk about his needs
with his wife without feeling too vulnerable, and talk
about his anxieties without feeling judged.

But what happens when the marriage is not providing continuity, an opportunity for parenting, emotional support, economic security, or open communication? Significant, continuous
symptom-producing stress is usually the result. The source of
the problem may not be simple to identify, but usually relates to
one or more of the following:

- a *crisis*, such as unemployment or the death of a child,
  which puts new demands on the marriage
- many *life changes* coinciding, such as a new baby join-
  ing the marriage just as a job transfer is moving your
  family across the country, resulting in confusion of roles
  and routines
- *individual needs* draining the ability of one or both
  partners to act like part of a team
- *role expectations* for your partner or yourself are so
  unrealistic that performance anxiety, resentment, or disappointment pushes out loving, caring feelings

For a marriage or family to survive such problems, it must be
able to change and reorganize itself. This runs counter to a
man's impulse during stress to maintain a sense of control by
holding fast to what is familiar. A husband may dream of how
things used to be instead of working toward how things might
become. A father may deny his child's changes instead of
exploring a new way of talking and listening. A retired man
may focus on a young lover, a new hairstyle, or a fresh social
life instead of identifying the depression he might be feeling.
But trying to take control over some changes is wasted energy.
Accepting change, perhaps with the help of a professional
counselor or therapist, may be more realistic.

Signs of marriage stress are not always clear. Fighting, yelling,
or sulking may be entirely absent, in fact. Consult the Marriage

Stress Checklist below for kinds of behavior that may be familiar to you. These examples can help you identify problems before they get out of hand.

MARRIAGE STRESS CHECKLIST

_____ I find that I am often annoyed at my wife or children for no reason.

_____ I suspect that I use my family as scapegoats for daily tension buildup.

_____ I act tough and unemotional even when I don't feel that way.

_____ I am least tolerant of behaviors of my wife or children that I dislike in myself.

_____ I often feel jealous or suspicious of my wife after I've had a fantasy about being unfaithful.

_____ I feel at a loss when my wife or children are upset.

_____ I often feel defensive, as if I am "walking on eggs," when I am at home.

_____ I often ignore problems with my wife in the hope that things will get better by themselves.

_____ I feel so guilty after being angry at my wife or children that I make it up to them by being overindulgent.

_____ I see my wife and children as extensions of me, and expect them to behave as I would behave.

_____ I find that I avoid going home by doing extra work at the office.

_____ I feel that I am not appreciated as a provider by my wife or family.

_____ I eat/smoke/drink compulsively when I come home at night.

_____ I have lost interest in being intimate or sexual with my wife.

_____ I frequently fall asleep and/or awaken earlier than I would like.

_____ I fear that I may become physically violent at home.

_____ I find it hard to think clearly when I am at home.

_____ I seem to have no sense of humor when I am at home.

_____ I feel as if I am "trapped" in my marriage.

_____ I feel lonely when I am with my wife and/or family.

Each item on this list reflects a possible cause or symptom of marital stress. Some items ask you to look at the ways in which you deal with yourself. If you are hard on yourself, you will probably be hard on your family. Some items ask you to look at your tendencies to avoid, deny, rationalize, or project problems. If you are doing this, you are probably experiencing some of the stress symptoms mentioned in the checklist. If you checked any one of the last ten items, discuss your feelings with your wife and consider professional counseling *together*. When there is marriage stress, the "patient" is the couple!

WHEN MARRIAGE FAILS

Social psychologist Zick Rubin of Brandeis University studied couples for two years and found surprising results. Although more women read romance novels and watch soap operas, men become infatuated with someone *more easily, more often,* and *with more serious consequences* than women. This means that more men than women marry for "love" rather than for practical reasons. This means that men are probably less likely to end marriages if they have an affair. In fact, after the third year of his study, Dr. Rubin concluded that men hold on to hope longer, are less likely to initiate separations, and suffer more than their partners in breakups.

Many men compound their stress during separation or divorce by seeing the process as a public display of failure. They often hide what they are going through from friends, co-workers, and relatives. This means they deny themselves possible sympathy, empathy, and company. If they feel guilty or ashamed, they further add to their stress by avoiding their children. In an attempt to preserve the "father figure," they may estrange or confuse their child. Children always want to know that *they* are not being divorced from their fathers, even though their mothers may be. Staying close and available to your children through a divorce may not be easy, but it is important for them and for you.

From my many interviews with men who are fathers not living with their children, three stresses emerged as most universal, though by no means most crucial:

Telephone Tension

If you find yourself worrying about your ex-wife picking up the telephone, worrying about choosing an interesting topic of conversation for your mid-week call to the children, or worrying about your own feelings of rejection in case your children again tell you that they are in the middle of a television show and can't talk—you have telephone tension.

Phone Phobia

If you find that every time the telephone rings you stiffen because you assume that the call must mean that your children are desperately ill or that your ex-wife is desperately broke—you have phone phobia.

Sunday Stress

If you find Sundays with the children stretching before you like an eternity, with only museums and bowling alleys available to fill the time—you have Sunday stress. Fathers do want to provide quality time when quantity is reduced, but are often overwhelmed at the prospect of supplying constant high-level entertainment. The answer is to provide interaction instead. You are Daddy, not Auntie Mame. Being together with your child is usually enough.

Less universal, but more crucial, is the divorced father's concern about another man entering his family's life. His ex-wife's boyfriend, husband, father, or brother may begin to have more contact with his children than he does. Country singer Mel Tillis called this other man "The Brand-New Mr. Me." In fantasy or reality, a divorced man with children feels his fatherhood threatened.

You can maintain your value as your children's father by *remaining* a father, rather than

- trying to be a buddy
- bribing them with gifts
- reversing roles so that they must parent you
- competing with their mother
- taking their emotional upheavals too personally
- withdrawing to test their love or loyalty

Don't stop seeing your children, even during the hard times. You were the first man in their life, and can never really be replaced. As difficult as it is to be a divorced father, it is still harder to be the child of divorced parents. Knowing what to expect, knowing what is happening, and knowing you are trying to do your best for you and your children can help all of you come through.

SEXUAL SURVIVAL UNDER STRESS

Since stress can distract, disorganize, depress, and depersonalize you, it can of course detour your sexual interest or functioning. Among women, the orgasm seems most vulnerable to stress; among men, the erection. This means that couples under stress may be finding their sex adding to their problems instead of helping to relieve their tension. Either partner may find that he or she is more frustrated after making love than before. Understanding the effect of stress on sexuality can provide a perspective and help prevent panic.

Recognize that stress increases a man's need for a sense of control, but that sex requires a relinquishing of many types of control. During sex, a man puts his pleasure in his partner's control; he trusts her to be in touch with his needs, and allows sensations to build until a reflexive orgasm occurs. "Letting go" in all three of these ways may be much more difficult for a man if he is holding on for dear life financially or occupationally.

Remember, as discussed in Chapter 3, that performance anxiety increases during stress, and that this decreases sexual responsiveness. Trying too hard, monitoring yourself, spectatoring, making up for failure in other areas, competing with your own past experiences, or attempting new records are counterproductive sexually. You can't take in pleasure when you are busy putting out self-conscious effort. Such stress distractions can either produce erectile problems or can insure premature ejaculation by allowing an orgasm to "sneak up" on you. Focusing on sensations, forgetting past and future, and feeling the fun of foreplay will help provide stress relief and sexual arousal.

A MEMO FOR THE WOMAN YOU LOVE

This section should be read by your wife or partner—together with you or on her own. It will help give you, as a couple, the means to survive sexually under stress. The first step is for your partner to examine some attitudes:

- Are you blaming yourself for your man's withdrawal or avoidance of sex? Don't. It is probably primarily his problem. If it was anger that led to erectile dysfunction, it is now his sexual problem, not his original anger, that is stressing him. If he is a victim of inhibited sexual desire, it is his depression that is probably keeping him there. But although it is his problem, it is your problem as well in that his stress interferes with your sexual functioning too. The situation calls for empathy rather than accusations or defensiveness. See a sex therapist together; let the "couple" be the patient, rather than insisting that he get help alone.

- Are you linking your self-esteem to his sexual response? Don't. Some feel if their husbands or partners don't respond to them sexually, they have failed personally. Again, this is probably much more his problem than yours. To check out the real factors involved, encourage him to check with his internist or urologist, and then see a sex therapist together.

- The next step is to help yourself and your mate relax sexually. Do your best to banish performance anxiety by creating an easy, nondemanding atmosphere. After all, orgasm is not the goal of sex play, it marks the *end* of sex play. Why rush?

- If you're in the mood for intimacy, take the initiative. You may be frightened by your mate's changing sexual capacities, but your mate is probably equally frightened and may be inclined to do nothing. If that is the case, the first move may have to come from you!

- Be prepared to try new styles of making love. Slower responsiveness may mean longer foreplay—which is certainly not bad news. Don't be afraid or ashamed to talk about what is going on. Your talking about your sex life may encourage your mate to do the same. In fact, you may both have been thinking the same things all along.

- Not everyone wants or needs to have an active sex life, but if you are one of those who do, enjoy!

MALE MID-LIFE CRISIS

It was Jack's fortieth birthday, but he didn't feel like celebrating. In the last seven days his grandfather and Frank, his closest childhood friend, had died. He and Frank had seen their first sexy film together. Jack's grandfather had been a strong man and Jack had felt he was indestructible. Now both were gone, and his birthday convinced him that he himself might be the next to go. He had never worried about aging before this. Today he did. He looked around and saw that his teenage son was the gorgeous guy the girls were looking at in the street. It made him feel proud and irritable at the same time. The "pretty boy" had become a middle-aged man.

Jack was experiencing many transitional stresses simultaneously. With the death of his grandfather, the composition of his family changed. With the death of his friend, a tie with his past was severed. With his decade birthday came a reassessment of his appearance. With the maturation of his son came Jack's shift to a different generational stratum. His son still had a grandfather, Jack did not. His son was a "hunk," Jack was not. Without fully realizing it, Jack had become a grown-up. Where was there to go after that?

Jack's answer was to go into a holding pattern for a year. He began to exercise and work out in a gym. This made him feel better about his body, used up some of the irritability he had been bringing home, and gave him a relief from competitive sports, which had begun to drain him. He then began to rethink his life pattern. He had always done what was expected of him. Now he asked what *he* expected of himself. He found that he wanted to change very little about his life pattern, but at least he started to feel that he was living it by *choice*.

Jack's experiences are not uncommon. Researchers using surveys, biographies, autobiographies, and case studies have come to similar conclusions about a man's stresses in his middle years. Whereas early adulthood stresses center around career and marriage decisions, later stresses do not seem to center around decisions at all. Later stresses seem to reflect an awareness that "do-overs" and "years to come" and "other chances" are less than realistic! Men in their middle years begin to realize that *this is their life.* Now. Not later.

Mid-life is the "noon of life," according to psychology pioneer Carl Jung, with the "afternoon and evening to come." The time when men awaken from The Dream. In *The Seasons of a Man's Life,* Daniel J. Levinson et al., remind us that success doesn't always lead to "happily ever after," and hard work may not even lead to success. Men become part of the "older generation" to their children, become "mentors" to employees and students, and become "responsible leaders" to their communities. This is their final chance to rechart or reconstruct their lives in a way that can still span decades.

With one foot in youth and the other in maturity, the middle years, then, are a time of readjustment for most men. Just like the mixed messages about manhood that cause so much male stress, the messages about a middle-aged man's future are mixed also:

- It will be a time to bask in public acclaim, or suffer public shame. This is when you will have made it or, if not, when you lost your shot.

- It will be the prime of life, or it will be the time you feel your age. You may find that you feel like a kid; or you may find that chronic disorders and stress symptoms have begun to take their toll.

- It's when you receive respect as an authority or elder; or it may be when you're seen as a tyrant, or "over the hill."

- It's a period when you can finally live for yourself; but you may find yourself alone because your wife or friends have died.

- It's a time when you can finally retire, or are forced to retire—the former with financial security, the latter with resentment.

- It's a chance for exciting creativity and leisure; or an eternity of boredom and apathy.

In other words, what is to come is largely unpredictable—which in itself, of course, creates anxiety. There is no clearly defined role from this point on. There is no assurance of health or wealth. Any man may be forced into retirement; may confront an economic recession, depression, or inflation when he is on a pension or social security; may be institutionalized or become dependent because of a stroke, heart condition, or other illness; may find himself isolated or his children's ward; may have to deal with the death of his child or even grandchild; may lose his sexual partner and feel guilty about sexual needs.

CAREER WORRIES AND RETIREMENT STRESS

"What is the meaning of life?" Sigmund Freud was asked. "Love and work" was supposedly his very direct and simple answer. If he was right, and man defines himself in terms of his work life and his love life, then the history of both will affect a man as he moves from manhood to maturity. If he is basically content with both, he is likely to see himself as having had a stimulating and fulfilled life. If he is basically discontented with both or either, he may have a sense of despair. As renowned psychologist Erik Erikson explained this, feeling like your one chance at life is drawing to a close may leave you bitter and resentful of those just starting out! The Male Stress Syndrome, then, does not end with middle age.

Careers, professions, and jobs usually have very different meanings to men. A *career* is an occupation that was *created* by a man. It has a personal history, which is his history. It is a unique history. A *profession* is an occupation that was *earned* by a man. He fulfilled requirements, studied, trained, and practiced. It is part of his identity. A *job* is an occupation that was *occupied* by a man. It is the way in which he made money and supported himself and his family. It is the work in his life, but not his "life's work."

The meanings of success, failure, and retirement are also very different for each type of work. A career is experienced by many as having a life of its own: a trouble-filled youth, an expansive, exhilarating "takeoff," a more steady or stable period, and then a sometimes subtle, sometimes sudden "falloff." Since stress increases as control, choice, and predictability decrease, careers can be highly stressful experiences even during successful periods! Unlike bureaucratic jobs, careers do not come with built-in security, job descriptions, sick leave, or retirement guarantees. High points may feel like fleeting, lucky interludes; low points may feel like personal failures. Retirement is too frequently the result of changing times rather than a man's choice.

> Henry started as a disc jockey for his college radio station in the Mid-west. Out of college, he took all the radio jobs he could find: station manager, engineer, cataloguer, time-checker, newscaster, and movie reviewer. Sometimes he got bored, sometimes he got fired. But he persisted because he was "entranced by the airwaves." He moved on to big cities, and often did well at finding spots for a few years at a time. His voice became known and his specialty became interviews. But he was always selling himself as his only product, and contracts were always up for review after eighteen months. By the time he was forty, he had four children and an ulcer. By the time he was fifty, his voice had become "too familiar" to be "fresh," and he was closed out of the airwaves. He now earns a good living in radio administration, but feels that his career is over.

Unlike Henry's career, Jack's profession offered more security. He knew what his options were when he graduated from dental school. He could teach dentistry, he could do a residency at a veterans' hospital, he could apprentice in a private practice and eventually buy in or buy the senior dentist out, he could form or join a dental group, or he could become associated with a medical group on a local, county, or state level. He worried about making the right choices at the right times; but unlike the career man, he was as much a consumer of a public need as he was consumed by the public. The more he practiced dentistry, the more his reputation grew. His successes did not feel like luck. His retirement would not be forced. When he did retire, he could probably even sell his practice for added financial security.

Where, then, is the stress for a professional man? In his constant sense of peer review. In his daily need to protect his license, reputation, or clients. In the demands that always exceed a workday. In the compromises that affect his wife and family: emergencies, office costs, and professional obligations. Like career success, professional success must be earned. This means many years of waiting for the "payoff"; and waiting, we know, can be one of the most difficult male stresses of all. And, finally, there is stress in retirement, which means a shift in identity. A man can't be a father without a son, or a husband without a wife, nor can he be a professional without a practice. After decades of defining himself as a doctor, dentist, or lawyer, he must now look at his daily life as a husband, father, or grandfather. His love life has now emerged over his work life to give his days shape. If the former was neglected or unsuccessful, the latter will be mourned and missed.

Jobs offer men yet a different set of stresses than do careers and professions. Men holding jobs may see themselves bypassed for new trainees, new machines, new or experimental job structures. New bosses mean old efforts no longer count. New accounts may mean more work, but new competition may mean industry unemployment. Sudden unemployment and forced retirement, in fact, put men at high risk for male stress symptoms. Studies suggest a four-time greater risk of depression and illness for men who had no choice about leaving their jobs than for men who voluntarily quit to change jobs or to retire. Again, that sense of loss of choice and control is activating the Male Stress Syndrome.

Why should forced retirement be so traumatic for any man, whether he be a career, professional, or workingman? For one thing, working makes you a productive member of society. You may be an "old hand," or a "veteran," but you are still paying your way. What are you when you retire? A "senior citizen," and that feels much different.

But that is just the beginning of the retirement stresses:

- You have lost the daily contact with co-workers. As bad as a job might be, as difficult as a career might be, or as demanding as a profession might be, co-workers can provide sympathy, humor, resources, and even emotional outlets. You can be fatherly, brotherly, or constructively critical and feel better afterward. At home alone, in your wife's domain, or within an institution, you may feel very lonely.

- You may experience boredom. Unless you have clear, workable ideas for your retirement, which are practical and which fit in with your family's plans as well, you may find that your retirement dreams were just that: dreams. You're not as likely to start projects and hobbies as you might be to continue activities that are part of lifelong interests that preceded retirement.

- You may find that you had equated your worth with your income. Now that you are living on pension or interest, you are feeling useless—unused, unnecessary, unwanted. Much of your identity was tied up in your occupation, and when that goes, so may a good measure of your morale. Bored, frustrated, not knowing what to do or expect of yourself, your sense of control can dwindle to the vanishing point. And stress grows proportionately.

  The way to avoid this is to retire *to* something. If you know when you're going to retire, plan in advance. If you're retiring because of illness, start planning while you're still in the hospital. If you can't seem to get started planning, if there seems to be nothing desirable you can realistically retire to, get counseling help as early as possible. You might never need it more.

  And, if you've had a dream about what you want to do when you retire, think seriously about implementing it. Don't dismiss it as something you're too old for. You're probably not too old at all. Giuseppe Verdi was in his eighties when he created some of his greatest operas. Pablo Picasso painted masterpieces into his nineties. And what about Michelangelo, Sigmund Freud, Frank Lloyd Wright, Colonel Sanders, Konrad Adenauer, and Charles de Gaulle?

• You may find that you are saddened by old memories, particularly if you are a widower as well as retired. Before you move to a new state, or even to a new building in your neighborhood, check it out carefully to make sure it has the conveniences, services, and lifestyle you need. Make sure it also has people you can relate to, groups you can join. This especially applies to moving from your own place to a retirement hotel, and it *most* especially applies to moving in with your children. Think very carefully—and, if you can, try the new situation out for a few months first.

If you're looking for something to do after you retire, marriage may give you an answer. But be sure it's the right one—give yourself a year or so after you retire before you make any permanent decision.

SUGAR DADDY VS. THE DIRTY OLD MAN

After decades of sexual activity, the older man is too often expected to leave such interests behind. Younger men may act as if they have discovered or invented sex and believe that no one over sixty could possibly feel the way they do. Cartoons depict sexuality in elderly men as laughable. Hospitals, institutions, and many nursing homes react to sexuality in the elderly as disgusting and inconvenient. If a much older man actively pursues women, actively seems interested in a sexual relationship, he's a "dirty old man." If he marries a much younger woman, he's a "sugar daddy" who is seen as foolishly being "taken" for his money. If he is a widower looking for a new wife, he is assumed to be looking only for companionship. If he is still married, even grown children picture their parents going into the sunset years hand in hand, not body to body.

In addition to social messages about his sexuality, the older man may have to deal with more tangible sexual setbacks. Strokes, diabetes, prostate problems, arthritis, cardiovascular illnesses, and disfiguring surgery may all mean some sexual loss, or enough embarrassment about body appearance that an older man may become more like a young teenager: sexual, but afraid to show his sexuality.

Recognizing the effects of aging on male sexuality is important so that physical changes will not frighten you or add to the stresses of the Male Stress Syndrome. With aging:

1. The "refractory" period, the period between an ejaculation and the time you can have your next erection, becomes longer. In youth, it can be as short as a few minutes; in older men it may last for hours.

2. The penis doesn't respond as readily to sexual images. Some men only have to fantasize to achieve an erection. With older men this usually doesn't happen. To obtain an erection they often need direct physical stimulation.

3. The penis may not become as hard or as full when it is erect. This may be due to a physical problem such as diabetes, a medication or drug, or natural changes over time.

4. There may also be less semen and a less forceful ejaculation. These have no practical effect on lovemaking, unless a man begins to worry about either.

Recognize that although there are changes in sexual functioning as a man ages, the main problem is usually the fear or worry that can stress him. As men become more aware of a loss in physical responsiveness, they often feel less manly and begin to avoid sex or check on themselves during foreplay. Once there is withdrawal or "spectatoring," sexual stress increases.

There are at least three good reasons for trying to counteract this potential for sexual stress. Sexuality helps all of us feel young, maintain a pleasure-filled relationship with our partner, and reduce stress through enjoyable exercise. In other words, it can be a physical and psychological minivacation from stress. And as an added bonus, some researchers suggest that sex may even help to relieve some symptoms of arthritis, since sexual arousal may stimulate increased production of cortisone by the body.

STRESS THROUGH THE SEVENTIES

As you continue to grow older, you're more likely to encounter two additional stresses: loss and the resulting isolation, and dependence on others.

LOSS AND ISOLATION

By the time you reach your seventies, both of your parents probably will have died. So may have other people who made up part of your life: other relatives, friends, acquaintances, tradespeople you spoke to, perhaps your wife.

These losses involve more than the stress of bereavement. They also leave you more alone. Especially if you lose your wife or anyone else you're living with, the isolation can be crushing; and if it keeps up it can lead to utter despair. Here are some guidelines to keep in mind:

- Don't move away if your wife dies and you've still got friends, or "friendly' institutions, in your neighborhood that you can call on or get to.

- Move away only if there's no place to go, nobody to talk to, where you are.

- Expand your interests. If you don't belong to a church or temple, join. If you do belong, join a committee.

- Take care of yourself physically. Exercise, watch your diet, and get regular health care.

- Start a long-term project. Plant some fruit trees. Buy

a pet. Study a new language, or take a course in computers.

Above all, if friends, relatives, or children offer to help, don't turn them away. It's not wise to give up your independence, but there's no need to deny yourself their company.

DEPENDENCE

At any age, illness can leave us physically dependent on others. After retirement, you may find yourself financially dependent on others. And as we grow older, we can all find ourselves in both conditions: physically *and* financially unable to give ourselves adequate care.

There are no easy answers, but there *is* a starting point for this stress management. As with a serious illness, the loss of independence is a *loss,* and should be treated as such. Expect to go through four stages of loss, whether the loss is a bereavement or a loss of independence or of a capacity.

Stage One: Denial
According to Milton Matz, a clinical psychologist and a former rabbi, step one in mourning usually involves denial. Some will avoid thinking or talking about the upsetting loss, some will go on with daily life pretending nothing has changed, and some will deny their emotions by becoming numb and unfeeling for a while.

Stage Two: Undoing
Magical thinking, which we all used as children, now often reemerges: make a wish, pick up sticks, count to five, hold your breath, give a large donation, eat special foods, go to sleep and when you wake up everything will be like it used to be. If the loss is a death, a man may attempt to substitute another person into the same role: remarry, or treat someone just like a son, or turn to another sibling. If the loss is one of a part of the body or a capacity, he may attempt feats or trips that are ill-advised.

Stage Three: Realization

Reality cannot be denied or side-stepped forever, and at some point a man will begin to feel his loss directly. Psychiatrist Elisabeth Kübler-Ross, world-famous for her research on death and dying, tells us that men most frequently say they turn to one of the following four sources of help when they face a crisis of loss:

- religious faith (God, church or synagogue, clergy)
- spouse (or other members of the family)
- themselves (contemplation, rationalization, understanding)
- physician (or psychiatrist or psychologist)

If he can find an answer to his question "What will life be like now?" a man can move on to Stage Four.

Stage Four: Rebuilding

Although life may be changed by a surgery, an illness, or a spouse's death, a man's value is not. If your father, grandfather, or friend is in the midst of rebuilding, you can help him recognize his value in the following ways:

- Seek out his company and share time with him even if it is quiet time or sad time.
- Listen to his pieces of plans without taking over for him. Taking over will not save him from anything. It will encourage him to feel useless or dependent.
- Try not to insist that he feel better about his loss. Telling him he is lucky to be alive after his heart attack, or that his wife was lucky that she died suddenly without pain, will not be startling news. It may, in fact, make him feel guilty about his anger, anxiety, or self-concern.
- Include him in as many of your plans as you can, but don't pressure him to accept. Letting him know that he is welcome and wanted is your aim.
- Show him as much affection as he can comfortably accept. Now is the time for a son to reassure his father

that he is loved and needed. Ask his advice, hug him, tell him that you care. Do it for your own sake as well as his. Provide your sons with this role model, and leave to yourself regrets about love left unsaid.

This last stage, rebuilding, may seem impossible to handle. What have you possibly got to rebuild with—or for? You still have yourself. Whatever was at the core of your being that held you together all these years hasn't deserted you yet. Whatever you've learned hasn't left you. These things still belong to you— and what belongs to you, you can share with others. And that's what you are rebuilding with, and what you are rebuilding for.

DEBUNKING MYTHS ABOUT THE MATURE MALE

Finally, if you are in the midst of your mature years now, here is some news that will encourage you and reduce the stress of anxious anticipation.

1. According to *myth*, as you grow older you lose some intellect. A number of studies that have followed thousands of people over several decades show that mental decline is *not inevitable* with aging. Dr. K. Warner Schaie, a psychologist at Pennsylvania State University, who followed more than 5,000 people over a thirty-five-year period, has found that there is less decline in those who have high verbal fluency, a successful career or other active involvement throughout life, and intellectual interests after retirement.

2. According to *myth*, older men lose interest in a sex life. According to Duke University psychologists George and Stephen Weiler, who studied 238 married men between the ages of fifty-six and seventy-one for a six-year period, four-fifths experienced *no* decline in sexual activity!

3. According to *myth*, the elderly are not a valuable commercial consumer group. According to conservative population projections, there will be more than 35 million Americans over the age of sixty-five by the year 2000.

4. According to *myth*, the elderly can expect senility. According to the statistics compiled by the U.S. Department of Health, Education and Welfare, and those available from the American Psychological Association, most of the symptoms that used to be grouped together as senility can now be identified as treatable symptoms of depression associated with poverty, chronic disease or pain, and institutionalization; or as specific symptoms of alcoholism or organic brain syndrome.

5. According to *myth*, elderly men can expect to find themselves abandoned by uncaring families. In 1990, elderly men were nearly twice as likely as elderly women to be married and living with their spouses (74 percent vs. 40 percent). The reality is that the majority of elderly men have a spouse for assistance, especially when health fails. Elderly widowed men have remarriage rates over eight times higher than elderly widowed women. According to the Policy Institute of the American Association of Retired Persons, over one half the elderly in their own households live within thirty minutes of a child; 13 percent are more than one hour away from a child; and 41 percent report daily contact with a child by telephone or in person.

6. According to *myth*, the greatest fear of the elderly is their own death. According to most research reports, older men are less concerned about dying than are younger men. Older men may feel pressure to make practical preparations in case of their death, but they tend to be realistic about its possibility and do not dwell on it.

Although male stress symptoms may be taking their toll in a man's later years, male stresses need not necessarily be increasing. As you will see in the next chapter, it is never too early or too late for stress management techniques.

9 LIVING WITH THE MALE STRESS SYNDROME

ALL MEN WILL FACE SOME STRESSES AND FEEL SOME STRESS SYMPTOMS DURing their lifetimes. This means that all men will encounter the Male Stress Syndrome. Understanding stresses and stress symptoms can be the starting point for managing male stress. Specifically, I am talking about saving or prolonging your life, your father's life, and the life of your son! The statistics and research in this area are clear: The time to start stress management is *today.*

Managing the Male Stress Syndrome starts, first, with knowledge and education. You must educate yourself about the differences between good stress (the kind over which you have some *choice, control,* and *predictability*, as outlined in Chapter 2), and bad stress (the kind you cannot control and which causes psychological problems and physical wear and tear on your body). You must familiarize yourself with the early warning signs of stress symptoms, as discussed in Chapter 3. You must learn how to assess your own stress risk and stress level, and you must learn coping techniques to reduce them both. Use the formula below to remind yourself of the cumulative effects of short-term and long-term stresses on your physical weak links, and of the possibilities of stress reduction that coping resources can offer:

short-term stresses + long-term stresses +
physical weak links – coping resources = stress risk

Short-term stresses would include emergencies such as a flat tire, a flooded basement, an unexpected snowfall, or a stalled subway; unpleasant experiences such as quarrels, unwelcome visits, or unreasonable requests; and temporary terrors such as rough airplane flights or evaluations by the boss.

Long-term stresses include most of the items on the now well-known life events scale (also called the Social Readjustment Rating Scale) developed by Thomas Holmes and Richard Rahe. Take a look at the scale that follows and add up the points shown for every item you've experienced in the past year; don't be thrown off by items that seem to apply to women only. (If your wife was pregnant, score yourself in that area as well.) Then check to see if your total point score falls into the low, moderate, or high stress-symptom-risk range. This will give you some idea of where your long-term stresses lie at the moment, and how much of an impact they have had on you in the past year.

SOCIAL READJUSTMENT RATING SCALE*

Life Event	Point Value
Death of spouse	100
Divorce	73
Marital separation	65
Jail term	63
Death of close family member	63
Personal injury or illness	53
Marriage	50

*Thomas H. Holmes and Richard H. Rahe, "The Social Readjustment Rating Scale," *Journal of Psychosomatic Research* 11 (1967), pp. 213–18.

Fired at work	47
Marital reconciliation	45
Retirement	45
Change in health of family member	44
Pregnancy	40
Sex difficulties	39
Gain of new family member	39
Business readjustment	39
Change in financial state	38
Death of close friend	37
Change to different line of work	36
Change in number of arguments with spouse	35
Mortgage or loan over $10,000	31
Foreclosure of mortgage or loan	30
Change in responsibilities at work	29
Son or daughter leaving home	29
Trouble with in-laws	29
Outstanding personal achievement	28
Spouse begins or stops work	26
Begin or end school	26
Change in living conditions	25
Revision of personal habits	24
Trouble with boss	23
Change in work hours or conditions	20
Change in residence	20
Change in schools	20
Change in recreation	19
Change in church activities	19
Change in social activities	18
Mortgage or loan less than $10,000	17
Change in sleeping habits	16
Change in number of family get-togethers	15
Change in eating habits	15
Vacation	13
Christmas	12
Minor violations of the law	11

YOUR TOTAL:

In their original sample poll in Seattle and from a later Navy study of 2,500 subjects, Holmes and Rahe found that people with scores over 300 points for one year had an 80 percent risk of becoming seriously ill or vulnerable to depression during the following year. Those with scores between 200 and 300 points still had an impressive 50 percent, or moderate, risk. Those with scores below 200 were at relatively low risk. Although these statistics cannot predict the risk for any particular individual, they do confirm the correlation between life-change stress and both physical and emotional health.

Long-term stresses also include behavior styles that make daily living more difficult. As we have seen, if you are a Type A or Type A+ man, you are potentially at higher risk for male stress symptoms than a man who practices Type B behavior patterns. Type A men *never* reach their goals—as soon as they approach one it becomes insufficient for them, and the next goal is set up!

Coping resources include stress identification (your ability to pinpoint stresses so that you can choose to confront them, flee from them, or at least diffuse their effects); exercise skills and relaxation techniques; and your support network, in all its different forms. Let's discuss each of these in turn.

STRESS IDENTIFICATION

Identifying your stresses early enough to prevent symptoms is an important management skill. Identification and recognition of stress permit you to get in there and *do* something, sooner rather than later. You may choose to confront the stressful situation, or you may choose to avoid it. You may choose to live through it and try to work off its effect through exercise or play. You may choose to neutralize its effects through relaxation. Or you may choose to change your attitude so as not to perceive the situation as stress.

The main point is that these options exist only *after* a stress has been identified. Without stress recognition, short-term stresses can become chronic long-term stresses that lead to the Male Stress Syndrome. Get to know your body signs of stress at their lowest levels. Intervene when you feel forehead muscles tightening; don't wait until you are wounded by a major headache. Intervene when you begin to feel rapid breathing; don't wait until you have hyperventilated or have frightening chest pains.

Get to know your particular psychological signs of stress as well. Are they some of the "six D's" listed in Chapter 3: defensiveness, depression, disorganization, defiance, dependency, or decision-making difficulty? Or are your signs behavioral? Do you become irritable, withdrawn, tired, agitated, jittery; compulsive about eating, smoking, drinking, or spending money? These behaviors are attempts at *distracting* yourself from stress. Distraction doesn't alter the original stress—it just adds a new one!

FIRST AID FOR SHORT-TERM STRESS

EXERCISE

Stress experts agree that exercise can be a vital coping resource. But which type of exercise should you choose? Jogging? Tennis? Aerobics? Isometrics? Swimming? Walking? The answer starts with the following question: Which type of exercise will you actually carry through? Three days of jogging will not help your body or your stress levels. A year of regular walks will! The exercise you choose should fit these parameters:

1. The type of exercise you choose should be approved by your physician after a physical examination and/or a stress test.

2. The exercise should not require unrealistic time or money expenditures. Traveling for an hour to and from an exercise club or paying large fees will quickly sabotage your exercise efforts.

3. The exercise should be realistically suited to your psychodynamics. If you are a competitive person, choose competitive one-on-one exercise. This will help you remain interested and motivated. If you are a team type, choose a league sport and enjoy the social activities that go with it. If you are not comfortable fighting for victory or having others rely on you, choose a self-regulated exercise routine and enjoy your time alone.

4. The exercise should ideally include a measure of improvement. This will give you an opportunity to achieve a sense of mastery: one more mile, one more push-up, one more run around the bases. An increased sense of mastery decreases a general sense of stress.

5. At least part of the exercise should include rhythmic repetition. Rhythmic activities relax our vigilance by following predictable patterns, and stress decreases as our rehearsal of a pattern increases. Running, counting, and chanting all leave us with no doubt as to what is going to come next. Just as the infant rocks himself to fall asleep and the young child asks to be told the same bedtime story again and again, the adult follows routines to give him a sense of control and security.

6. The exercise, though it may be rhythmic, should not be mindless. Some concentration on the activity means some distraction from stress. Exercise time can be time out from daily demands and mental lists. By focusing on your workout, you are narrowing your world to a very manageable size. For the moment, at least, nothing else matters but your body and its movements.

7. The exercise you choose should be strenuous enough to use up stress-induced adrenaline without leaving

you exhausted. The body's stress reaction is suited for fight or flight. If you have been stuck behind a desk all day, this adrenaline is doing you little good and probably a lot of harm. Make use of it in a constructive, controlled, stimulating way, or it will make you irritable, jittery, and tense.

8. If you are using exercise as part of a weight control program, schedule it for mornings. Unfortunately, exercise itself does not keep you thin—six hours of tennis would reduce your weight by only one-half pound! But exercise does seem to reset your metabolism at a higher level for almost twelve hours, and it also seems to reset your appestat at a lower level for many hours. Exercising in the morning, then, will help you eat less and burn more calories during the day, according to internist Leonard Lustgarten of New York's Lenox Hill Hospital.

Although brisk walking is the common aerobic exercise for men and women of all ages, jogging has been popular among men who want more of an aerobic workout for their hearts. Exercises designed to strengthen the cardiovascular and respiratory system come in many other forms as well: swimming, biking, jumping rope, and using a treadmill—but they are all called aerobic because they aim to increase the supply of oxygen to the muscles. These exercises leave you not so much with aches and pains in your muscles, but with labored breathing and pounding heart. You know the exercises are working when for a given level of exertion you are breathing easier and your heart isn't pounding as hard. Check with your physician for the appropriate aerobic exercise plan for you and follow these guidelines:

• Don't start or stop exercising suddenly. Always warm up slowly and gradually taper off your activity to give your blood pressure and muscles an opportunity to adjust to the demands of the exercise.

- Build up your cardiovascular system gradually. Walking one mile in about fifteen minutes, four or five times a week, is usually enough to increase the blood supply to the heart. This means fewer beats per minute will be needed and the heart, therefore, will be less taxed.

Health club members, which include almost 20 percent of men between twenty and forty-four years of age, usually combine muscular endurance exercises with isometrics and isotonics. Muscular endurance exercises are calisthenics, well suited to music faster than your heartbeat of seventy-two beats per minute. Isometric exercises involve the use of force against an immovable object or resisting set of muscles. Isotonic exercises strengthen muscles through weight-lifting. These exercises, like aerobics, require a warm-up period first, in which stretching and flexing movements gradually increase blood flow to the muscles and redirect your attention from other concerns to your exercise.

Sometimes it is not possible to use exercise as an aid for stress. Relaxation techniques may be used instead to redirect your attention from stress. These techniques will shut off the adrenaline output rather than use it up.

MEDITATION AND DEEP RELAXATION

There's some controversy about whether there is a difference between meditation and deep relaxation; but there's little doubt that whatever it's called, it's doing people good. What both meditation and deep relaxation amount to is shutting the world off, slowing your internal clock, and detaching yourself from your worries and preoccupations, for at least ten minutes to half an hour. If you can do that by sitting alone in a chair in a darkened room, then that's all you need.

One of the advantages of meditation techniques is that they're organized. They give you a definite routine to follow and tell you how to handle distractions. Practice the exercises and, probably within a month, you'll be able to glide into relaxation.

According to Eric Eckholm, reporting in *The New York Times*, meditation produces:

- lower metabolism
- lower muscle tension
- slower heartbeat
- slower breathing
- lower blood lactate levels (a chemical associated with anxiety)

In other words, meditation seems to reverse stress responses.

Autohypnosis

Autohypnosis is self-suggested relaxation. Stanley Fisher, a New York psychologist who specializes in teaching autohypnosis, recommends the following exercise for relaxation and stress intervention. It's also a good remedy for insomnia, and it's not hard to do.

1. Sit comfortably in a chair facing a wall about eight feet away. Pick a spot or an object on the wall that is about one foot above your sitting eye level. This is your focal point.

2. Look at your focal point, and begin counting backward from 100, one number for each breath you exhale.

3. As you count and continue to concentrate on your focal point, imagine yourself floating, floating down, down through the chair, very loose and relaxed.

4. As you stare at your focal point you will find that your eyelids feel heavier and begin to blink. When this happens, just let your eyes slowly close.

5. While your eyes are closed, continue to count backward, one number for each time you exhale. As you count, imagine how it would feel to be as limp as a rag doll, totally relaxed and floating in a safe, comfortable space. This is your space. Furnish it in any way you choose.

6. As that safe, comfortable feeling flows over you, you can stop counting and just float.

7. If any disturbing thought enters your space, note it and just let it flow out again; continue to feel safe and relaxed.

8. Set your internal alarm for five minutes (although you could choose to stay longer).

9. When you're ready to come out of autohypnosis, either let yourself drift off to sleep, or count from one to three and exit using the following steps: At one, let yourself get ready; at two, take a deep breath and hold it for a few seconds; and at three, exhale and open your eyes slowly. As you open your eyes, continue to hold on to that relaxed, comfortable feeling.

My favorite autohypnosis routine takes about two minutes of your busy time. Try it three times each day. While you are seated at your desk or on a bus or on the side of the bed, place your hands comfortably in your lap, both feet on the ground, and focus on a faraway spot at eye level.

1. Count backward from ten to one slowly, taking a breath on each count, and then exhaling leisurely.

2. Allow your eyes to close. Again count backward from ten to one, taking a breath on each count, exhaling leisurely, and allowing tension to flow out of your body as you exhale.

3. With your eyes still closed, count backward from ten to one again. This time, imagine that your breath is a mist of color. Every time you exhale, you will be creating more and more of a cloud from this mist.

4. Float in this mist until your eyes open by themselves.

Try to add an extra count of ten each week until you reach fifty, rather than thirty as described above. By providing rhythm (counting), slowing respiration, and distracting you from stress by utilizing imagery, this routine is a highly effective stress reducer.

Progressive Relaxation

This simple formula is often taught to children during their rest period at nursery school. It works for adults, too.

1. Starting with your toes, relax them.
2. Then the feet and ankles: relax.
3. Then the calves: relax.
4. The knees: relax.
5. The thighs: relax.
6. The buttocks: relax.
7. The abdomen and stomach: relax.
8. The back and shoulders: relax.
9. The hands: relax.
10. The forearms: relax.
11. The upper arms: relax.
12. The neck: relax.
13. The face: relax.
14. Drift off . . .

Progressive Muscular Tension/Relaxation

This exercise has two benefits. In the short run, it helps you relax your muscles. In the long run, if you keep at it, it sensitizes you to recognizing your body's tensions, so you can do something about them before they become painful or chronic.

1. Frown as hard as you can for ten seconds; then relax those forehead muscles for ten seconds. Now repeat this more quickly, frowning and relaxing for one second each and becoming aware of the different feelings of each movement.
2. Squeeze your eyes shut for ten seconds, then relax for ten seconds. Repeat quickly.
3. Wrinkle your nose hard for ten seconds; then relax for ten seconds. Repeat quickly.

4. Slowly press your lips together; then relax. Repeat quickly.

5. Press your head back against the wall, floor, or bed (real or imaginary)—then relax. Repeat quickly.

6. Bring your left shoulder up in a tight, shrugging motion; relax. Repeat quickly.

7. Do the same with your right shoulder; repeat quickly.

8. Press your straightened arms back against the wall or floor or bed; relax. Repeat quickly.

9. Clench your fists tightly for ten seconds. Relax your hands and let the tension flow out through your fingers. Repeat quickly.

10. Contract your chest cavity for ten seconds and re-ease. Repeat quickly.

11. Press your back against the wall or floor; relax. Repeat quickly.

12. Tighten your buttock muscles for ten seconds; relax. Repeat quickly.

13. Press your straightened legs against the wall or floor or bed; relax. Repeat quickly.

14. Slowly flex your feet, stretching your toes as far back toward you as possible; relax and let tension flow out through your toes. Repeat quickly.

15. Check for tense spots and repeat the exercise where you find any.

REMEDIES FOR INSOMNIA

Many preparations that put you to sleep also tend to disturb your natural sleep rhythms, so they may not be the best thing for you. If you've had a stressful day, the time to tackle insomnia is a few hours before your usual bedtime.

1. *Don't eat a heavy meal*; in fact, cut down on the solid

food and drink extra liquids. The idea is to rest your digestive system and let other parts of your body start healing themselves.

2. *Stay away from caffeine*—coffee, tea, chocolate, and most soft drinks. This sounds too obvious to mention, but many people think that one cup of coffee won't affect them. It will for about six hours. Just before you go to bed, drink a glass of warm milk, instead. Mom was right; it really may help you fall asleep. Milk contains L-tryptophan, which scientists have found to be a mild natural sedative. So if you are milk-tolerant, try it.

3. Don't get into bed until you're *sleepy*—or you'll get used to being wide awake while you're in bed.

4. Keep the room cool, keep it quiet, and keep it dark, because warmth, noise, and light trick your body into responding as if it were morning. Actually 65° is ideal for sleeping because while warmth might make you fall asleep, a cool temperature helps you stay asleep.

5. *Give yourself time to relax, especially to laugh.* And try one of the simple relaxation techniques described earlier in this chapter.

BIOFEEDBACK

Biofeedback uses machines or computers to feed back to you specific changes in your body's functioning that are ordinarily too subtle for you to pick up before damage is done. The most common functions are muscle tension, pulse rate, temperature of your extremities, and brain wave activity. Generally, an electronic sensor is attached to you (usually by wrapping; there's no pain or discomfort at all), and immediately a signal is produced. This is typically a clicking sound, but it could be flashing lights.

If the clicks slow down, it means that the activity (heart rate, say) is slowing down; if the clicks speed up, the activity (hand temperature, say) is always rising. After a while, you recognize early signs of these "automatic" activities and can bring them under your voluntary control. Soon you will be able to moderate them at will without the machine. You will notice your heart rate increasing much earlier on, and you will notice changes in your skin temperature before your head begins to pound. This allows you to switch to a more relaxed mode. Biofeedback is useful, among other things, for controlling migraines, hypertension, some heart arrhythmias, and gastrointestinal disorders. Many clinics and health-related facilities offer biofeedback training.

SOOTHING ENVIRONMENTS

Set up soothing environments for your body and your mind. Your body can be soothed by a warm bath, a steamy shower, or five minutes of shut-eye in the sunshine coming in through the office window. Charles Crowley, a professor of criminal justice, recommends a quick lunchtime nap on a lightweight, inexpensive webbed lawn chaise that can be folded away behind your file cabinets. Robert Salzman, an attorney, recommends a living-room chair set up to face a plant and surrounded by favorite books and magazines just waiting to be read. Ernest Collebolleta, a high-school teacher, recommends floating, not swimming, in body-temperature water at the nearest YMCA or health club.

Your mind can be soothed by mental vacations from daily details such as browsing through a bookstore (from the do-it-yourself section to the fiction department), listening to music (music with a beat slower than your heartbeat—seventy-two beats per minute—tends to be relaxing), or even planning a new construction (bookshelves, deck, or toy box). Completing the plans may be relaxing, too; but it's not necessary. And don't forget fishing, films, and having fun with your children. Michael Braverman, a real-estate developer, recommends spending some time every day looking at the horizon to help you realize how much more there is to life beyond your daily problems. These are both mental and physical escapes that turn off the stress system.

REORGANIZE FOR RELAXATION

Clean out the garage, rearrange your tool chest, or set up a new tax record sheet. Any act of organization will increase your sense of control. As your sense of control increases, your sense of stress will decrease. It seems that the pituitary gland doesn't distinguish between settling a major crisis and straightening out a cluttered attic. Either is a job well done, thus shutting off the adrenaline output for a while.

PLAY

Don't send your children out to play—join them. It's good for all of you. Play games like backgammon for distraction, games like cards for socializing, and games like scrabble for self-improvement. Play games with teams if you enjoy the camaraderie, or one-on-one games if you enjoy the competition. And if you are competing, compete openly. That way, you give yourself permission to celebrate victory if you win and to demand a rematch if you lose.

LONG-TERM STRESS-MANAGEMENT TECHNIQUES: HELPING OTHERS

Women have a long history of helping each other. They take each other to the doctor, console each other's losses, celebrate each other's joys, act as midwives for each other, and often share the widowhood years together. Men, unfortunately, do not typically have this helping history. They do share sports, fights, fun, and drinks; they even complain to each other. But they do not ask each other for help. As I have said before, male fears and tears get hidden, not helped. Now is the time to begin to change this pattern. Your son needs you. Your father needs you. Your friends may need you. Your wife or lover or mother may need you too, in a way that may be new to you.

Here are some suggestions for stress crisis management. You are not being asked to be a therapist or social worker. Rather, you are being introduced to some techniques that will help you help others to help *themselves.* Furthermore, you will be helping your son to see you as a nurturer as well as a provider, and helping your father to see you as a son who can give to him as well as take from him. It might not be easy for your son or father to allow you to help them. After all, they have had the same grin-and-bear-it training you have had. So you may become a new role model as well as a new coping resource for them!

First, become aware of the major male stresses that statistics tell us trigger severe physical and/or psychological stress symptoms.

Second, be aware of the signs of male stress at a crisis level: unusual emotional swings with disorganized and confused behavior, dramatic reduction of work and social functioning, sleep and eating disturbances due to anxiety or depression.

Third, be firm about professional intervention when stress is at a crisis level. Michael Hoyt, a psychologist at Kaiser Permanente Medical Center in Hayward, California, warns that professional help is indicated if a man or woman reports:

- feeling overwhelmed
- feeling trapped
- having suicidal impulses
- having homicidal fantasies or impulses
- turning to alcohol or drugs

If stress is not at one of these emergency levels, or if you must wait before professional help is available, I recommend the following plan, which was first presented in *The Female Stress*

Syndrome. It embodies family counseling, stress management, and crisis-intervention techniques developed by psychologists throughout the past decade.

1. Look for the *"six D's."* They will let you know that a man feels stressed.
    *   *Dependency* needs are increased (though he might deny or try to hide it).
    *   *Decision-making* is difficult—even simple decisions about clothes or food.
    *   *Depression* influences his outlook and dominates his emotions.
    *   *Disorganization* and even panic are reflected in his daily behavior.
    *   *Defensiveness* makes him argumentative and sensitive.
    *   *Defiance* can interfere with his work and family relationships.

2. Show him that you *care.* Even if you share his alarm, do not show it—express concern instead. Try to understand the stress from his point of view, not your own. In this case the reality is not as important as the experience. Here are some things you might say:

    "I want to understand what you're going through."

    "I'm glad to have a chance to spend some time with you."

    "Have you ever gone through this kind of thing before?"

3. Encourage him to *talk* about his problem. Talking gives him a sense of "doing" something. Talking gives him an opportunity to "hear" himself, "listen" to himself as he would to another. Try saying:

    "Tell me a little more about this."

    "How do you explain that?"

    "I'm not clear about . . ."

    "What have you done that made you feel better (worse)?"

4. Be what psychologist Carl Rogers calls an *active listener*. Rogerian psychologists would recommend that you repeat what your friend or relative has said as a check for accuracy, and repeat what you have heard to reassure him that you have really been listening. Also, repeat with warmth and sympathy to indicate that you accept the feelings being shared with you.

    "What I hear you saying is . . ."

    "I think I understand. You feel as if . . ."

    "You certainly seem to think . . ."

    "Do you mean . . ."

5. Help him *help himself*. Taking over for him will only increase his sense of being overwhelmed, helpless, and out of control. Taking over will interfere with any learning that might otherwise result from managing a stress experience. To increase his self-help capabilities, follow the rest of the steps outlined.

6. Ask for a plan of action. Assess the risk-reward ratio. Discuss alternatives.

    "How do you plan to . . ."

    "What do *you* plan to do?"

    "Did you ever think that you might also try . . ."

7. Work on his *fine-tuning*. That is, help him to focus on the problem without blurring the picture with exaggeration, anxiety, or anticipation. Sort the facts from the fictions.

    "From what you're telling me, it seems . . ."

    "Let me see if I can say that another way . . ."

    "What's the most practical way to go about this?"

    "If you decide to do that, then you'll probably also have to . . ."

8. Develop a *contract* for a specific course of action. This accomplishes two stress-management goals. It makes his responsibility for self-help clear, and it gives him a chance to increase his self-esteem by carrying through a plan during a stressful time.

"So by Wednesday, you're going to . . ."

"Now, I'm counting on you to . . ."

9. *Recapitulate* as often as necessary, since your friend or relative is likely to be easily distracted.

"Now, you told me that you'd . . ."

"Let's make sure we know what we're doing . . ."

"Tell me again what you're going to do next."

10. Provide a *safety net*. Discourage withdrawal from friends and family or support systems. Encourage him to develop a network of resource people—informal "hot lines."

"Remember, I'll be around tonight at six and tomorrow at . . ."

"Let's get together again tomorrow (Wednesday, etc.) . . ."

"Who're you planning to spend the evening (weekend, holiday, etc.) with?"

11. Set up *structure*. We all do better when we are not at loose ends or with time on our hands. Mourning rites (wakes, shivas, etc.), baptisms, confirmations, bar and bat mitzvahs, and even weddings can provide structure during periods of transition or stress. Make use of such social institutions.

12. There are cases in which we are dealing with a problem that cannot truly be "solved" (one-sided love, fatal or chronic illness, etc.). In these cases, promote appropriate *acceptance*. This will help reduce useless persistence and directionless activity; and it will help reduce the effects of the Male Stress Syndrome.

HELPING YOUR FATHER

Your father may need different kinds of help at different ages. The following advice touches on many of these areas:

- Take him seriously. You don't have to agree with him,

you can argue with him as much as you want; but don't simply dismiss him and his opinions.

- Accept his sexuality—and his girlfriends.

- Encourage him to talk about his changed status. You don't have to offer any advice; just let him talk. Being with his family, talking out his fears, anger, and resentment, will help him find his own way out of emotional problems.

- Let him be generous if he wants to. He's not trying to control you; he's trying to control his own situation. And if he's cheating himself on one or two material things, he's rewarding himself enormously with enhanced feelings of usefulness.

- Encourage him to remain independent as long as he'd like. At the same time, begin to include him more often in family outings. Respect his refusals, but don't stop asking.

- If he needs a caretaking institution, let him join in the selection process. The financial and physical burden of supporting a chronically ill father in his home or yours can be heavy, and you shouldn't have to bear it indefinitely. But give him some voice in his destination. Visit him often. And take him (and his friends, if possible) on frequent excursions away from the home.

Remember, he'll be struggling to maintain his dignity and not give way to despair. You can make all the difference in the world.

LONG-TERM STRESS-MANAGEMENT TECHNIQUES: HELPING YOURSELF

Always remember, as I said in *The Female Stress Syndrome* as well, that *you are entitled to try to reduce the stress in your life*. Give yourself permission to take control over your life, to have and to express feelings, and to separate your past from your present.

Don't re-create old scenarios again and again with the new people in your life. They will not change in the reliving. They will not give you mastery over the past. Instead, address the present: it is only the present over which you can really take control.

Why assume the future will be the same as the past? Our view of the past is never objective anyway. Our earliest introduction to the world leaves a lasting impression, it is true; however, this first impression can be sorted out from the different reality of the present. The child's point of view in each of us can be recognized by us, tolerated with self-understanding, and then redirected and guided by the adult in us.

CULTIVATE SUPPORT NETWORKS

What is a support network? In its simplest form, it consists of people you can talk with. And why is talking so important for stress management?

1. Talking about a problem or stress gives you a chance to *hear yourself*. You can listen to yourself more calmly when you are saying something aloud than when you are thinking it alone in the middle of the night. In trying to explain your stress to another, you often clarify it for yourself as well.

2. Talking with someone reminds you that you are not alone. Someone cares enough to listen—someone who can probably sympathize and tell you that he or she, too, has had similar stress.

3. Talking it out can replace impulsive acting out. Sometimes neither fight nor flight are real solutions to stress, even though they are our first responses. Talking feels like a form of action. It is a first step in doing something about a stressful situation—a step that

leaves many second steps open as options.

4. Talking to someone you respect can lead to useful feedback and suggestions—perhaps a new perspective that will permit you to view the stressful situation less personally, defensively, or irately. Perhaps talking to someone will give you a different attitude toward what you can expect from yourself or from others.

5. Talking alerts others to your needs, and gives them a chance to share their resources with you. You now have *their* network, as well as your *own*, at your disposal.

Who constitutes part of a support network? Potentially all the people in your life. Check the list below to see how many of these people you talk with when you are under stress:

____ mate (wife, lover)
____ friends (male or female)
____ parent (mother, father, both)
____ older children (son, daughter)
____ brother(s)
____ sister(s)
____ co-workers
____ clergy
____ physician
____ therapist (psychologist, psychiatrist, social worker, etc.)

Now review the list again and focus on those you did *not* check. Can any of these people be added to your support network? If you are experiencing stress in some area and feel that there is no one you can talk to, jump to the end of the list and contact a professional as soon as possible. Remember, according to a University of California study, men without a good support network have *double* the health problems of others after a stressful event, and are *three times* as likely to suffer from depression.

USE "AS-IF" TECHNIQUES

If you expect the worst, it often comes to be—in part because you are behaving with anticipatory anxiety, creating tension, and getting stressed responses from others. Psychologists call this a negative self-fulfilling prophecy. That is, you predict disaster, behave accordingly, and thus contribute to making your fears come true.

Roger was engaged to Diane. He loved her and wanted to marry her, but spent night after night suspecting that she would pull out of the relationship before the wedding. "I'm not as good-looking as she is, or as young," he'd ruminate. "Why is she marrying me? Money? Security?" He began to monitor her words, looking for hidden meanings. He began to check on her appointments to reassure himself that they were not rendezvous. He began to withdraw sexually to test her devotion, and to complain of financial problems to test her motives. He soon succeeded only in convincing her that he no longer loved her, and she did pull out of the engagement. Roger felt his worst fears were confirmed, became more suspicious than ever, and never examined his own role in breaking up the engagement—or his motives for doing so!

If you are inclined to create negative self-fulfilling prophecies to protect yourself from disappointments, *stop*. All you are doing is adding your own insult to injury, plus increasing the risk of the Male Stress Syndrome by mixing in some anticipatory anxiety with real stresses that cannot be avoided. Expect the best, instead. Even if "the best" does not materialize, at least you have eliminated stress before the problem or disappointment.

Counter your negative vicious circle with the "as-if" technique. Behave "as if" everyone will naturally treat you just the way you want to be treated.

John was an engineer, but his training had been in Europe. His father was in the military and John had not been in the United States for two decades. Now he was back and job hunting. He needed a certain level of income to meet his family obligations, but felt that his foreign degree and experience might be overlooked. He was prepared for criticism and rejection, and found that he was procrastinating about job hunting. His situation was becoming desperate. He finally decided to try the "as-if" technique. He entered interviews "as if" he had been educated here and presented himself "as if" he were a valuable catch for anyone fishing for an employee. He found that his resistance to making interview appointments let up and that his interview manner became more relaxed, open, and friendly. He, of course, landed a job quickly. He might have eventually anyway, but with much procrastination, anticipatory anxiety, and stress!

As I point out to both my male and female clients and patients, the "as-if" assumptions are usually closer to reality than the pessimistic ones. Furthermore, this technique makes it more easy to:

- ask for favors without defensiveness
- teach others that we see ourselves as worthwhile and entitled to positive treatment
- express feelings without anticipatory anger
- flatter others by making *requests*, not demands
- influence reactions in others that will reduce, not increase, our stress

Negative prophecies sabotage your own efforts to communicate by broadcasting expectations of disappointment, by broadcasting criticism and resentment. Try positive self-fulfilling prophecies and help yourself reduce the Male Stress Syndrome.

CHANGE YOUR MIND

Not constantly, not whimsically, not irresponsibly; but whenever new information or time to think leads you to new conclusions. Too many men have told me that they fear losing the respect of their children, wives, co-workers, or friends if they "back down" from a position they have taken in the past. But such attempts at rigidity will only aggravate stressful situations by putting you into conflict with your own feelings.

Some men handle this problem by giving themselves plenty of time before making any public statement about their decisions. They say to their children, "Let me think about that." They say to their wives, "You have a point. Let's talk more later."

They say to their bosses, "I'll have to get back to you on that."

Some men offer their opinions and decisions quickly, but add, "That is how I feel right now."

Some men state both sides of any issue and play devil's advocate to give themselves psychological room for a change of mind.

Some men have taught themselves to change their minds with explanations, not excuses; firmly, not tentatively, and without self-judging. One seventy-nine-year-old patient has told me, "I always allow myself to change my mind—it's my proof that I still have one!"

ENJOY YOUR SEXUALITY

Like compulsive eating, drinking, or drug abuse, compulsive sexual behavior in any form is a stress symptom. If you find that you are trying to relieve all your stresses through sexual encounters or masturbation, consult a sex therapist or psychotherapist. He or she can help you better define your stresses and find more specific types of solutions appropriate to your problems.

If, on the other hand, you find that your stresses are leading you to be less interested in sex, remember this: by becoming performance-focused or orgasm-oriented, too many men add stress to an activity that can potentially *reduce* stress. Sex can narrow your world, temporarily, to a private and cozy one. It can remind you that you are needed and wanted, that you are able to give someone pleasure and that you are able to make someone feel like giving you pleasure. It can be a time when you take in good feelings and sensations rather than irritation and stress. It can leave you feeling desirable, attractive, comforted, relaxed, and bonded rather than alone.

UNDERSTAND ANGER

Men may find it easier to become angry than women do, because anger is not one of the "weak" emotions. But many men do have a conflict about anger nevertheless, because to them it represents a loss of emotional control. Some fear that they may lose control if they lose their temper; and control is the one thing they don't want to lose. Some are afraid of what their anger can do to others, so they hold it in.

But it is important to express anger in order to save your heart, and it's possible to do it without losing control or alienating the important people in your life.

1. Understand that what you want to express is your own hurt or anger. Don't confuse these feelings with power plays, vengeance, or anything else. Your message to the other person is, "I am angry" or "I am hurt." It should *not* be, "You are terrible" or "I'm gonna get you." Unfortunately, many of us are trained, in a sense, to express anger in terms of abuse or threats. So we'll shout at somebody we love, "You're the stupidest person in the world"; or, at somebody we wouldn't dream of hurting, "I'd like to wring your neck." We don't really mean it, but it doesn't seem that way to the other person. So stick to the basic message.

2. Don't generalize; talk about the specific incident that upset you. If your wife forgot to shut off the hose, stay with that; don't generalize into "She's always forgetting to shut off the hose" and then into "She always forgets everything." (If she *is* always forgetting to shut off everything, then that's something to be discussed in a calm, problem-solving manner, to negotiate or get help with —not something to keep losing your temper about.) So don't wander into side issues, a tendency that is called "kitchen-sinking"—that is, throwing everything into the argument. Keep the anger localized.

3. Finally, if the other person offers an explanation, *listen*; and if the other person offers an apology, *accept*. The main thing is: You're not out to win points, you're out to get rid of the anger; so let the incident end as soon

as possible. And again, if it keeps on happening, getting angry isn't going to change it. (It hasn't changed it yet, has it?) But a calm, friendly discussion might help—*after* you're over your anger.

SWITCHING OFF TYPE A BEHAVIOR

I've described Type A behavior in some detail earlier, so here I will just summarize its basic features:

- irritability
- impatience
- aggravation
- hostility
- overscheduling
- perfectionism
- polyphasic behavior (doing more than one thing at a time)

These are not features you're born with. They're part of a learned way of coping with the need to achieve, to be aggressive, and to be in control that is instilled into men almost from birth. And because Type A behavior is something you learn, or teach yourself, it's also something you can *un*learn. It's not easy, but there's nothing more rewarding. It has two big payoffs: a longer life for you and better relationships with those you love.

The switch requires work in three areas: awareness, substitution, and reinforcement.

Awareness

Awareness involves what I call the three "R's": recognition, re-evaluation, and remediation. *Recognize*, from minute to minute, the stressors that trigger physical or behavioral symptoms in you. This must be done as stress is building, not after it's left you limp.

Then *re-evaluate* the importance of these stressful demands, which are being imposed on you by others or by yourself. Take yourself off automatic pilot and rebuild your energy budget from the bottom up. Make a choice, from minute to minute, about every activity in your day, and set priorities; do this day after day. And resolve not to overschedule, no matter how important it seems.

Finally, identify stress remedies that work for you. Perhaps it's relaxation, which shuts off the body's emergency response system. Or perhaps it's exercise, which uses up the adrenaline that's been pouring into your blood all day. This is the aspect of *remediation*, mopping up the stress effects that have infiltrated your body.

Substitution

Eliminate a part of your life and you've left a vacuum. Unless that vacuum is filled, the behavior you've banished will come sneaking back again. That's where Part Two comes in: the deliberate substitution of low- or no-stress behavior for high-stress behavior.

- Substitute sit-down meals for sandwiches on the run—and try to make these knife-and-fork meals.

- Substitute a hobby—*any* hobby—for working overtime consistently.

- Substitute a non-competitive sport such as swimming, jogging, or simply walking for one of your competitive tennis matches this weekend. Or if you're captain of the bowling team, think of dropping down voluntarily to a less stressful playing position.

- Substitute some playtime with your children tonight instead of clearing up paperwork at your desk or at home.

- Substitute lovemaking with your wife for "helpful hints" on how she should handle her own work.

- Allow yourself the time to walk, talk, and drive more slowly. Soon your heart will beat more slowly also, and your age will show less rapidly.

Reinforcement

Reinforcement, or feedback, is a vital part of any behavior-modification plan. Positive reinforcement means giving yourself a reward; negative reinforcement means giving yourself a reprieve from punishment. Both can help you make the switch away from Type A behavior.

Deliberately reward yourself whenever you recognize, re-evaluate, and remediate a stressful situation. How?

- Give yourself a dollar toward something you want to buy.
- Give yourself fifteen minutes' extra sleep on the weekend.
- Give yourself a fifteen-minute session listening to music slower than your heartbeat (slower than seventy-two beats per minute).
- Give yourself thirty minutes toward planning a trip you've always wanted to take.
- Think of your own rewards, or talk the situation over with your wife or family. Maybe you can come up with some joint rewards that can make everybody happier.

Substitutions and rewards can help you cope with stressful situations, or ease your ulcer, or stimulate your sense of humor, or rid you of your headache. These substitutions and reinforcements are reminders that while it feels good to stop banging your head against a wall, it feels better not to start. Both will also encourage you to take control over your stressful behaviors and demands. Don't wait until it's too late!

USE HUMOR

If there's one stress remedy that's probably as good as all the others combined, it's laughter. Laughter is a signal for the body's emergency response system to turn off. It relaxes the facial muscles, lowers the body armor, restores perspective—and helps others do the same. So it also defuses stressful situations. It's the best possible civilized response to the fight or flight syndrome; and, according to Norman Cousins's book *Anatomy of an Illness,* it can even promote healing. So next time you feel under stress, take two jokes and call a friend in the morning. He'd like to hear them too.

TAKE CONTROL OF YOUR LIFE

Men are brought up to value control, and that can be a major contributor to stress. But it doesn't have to do us harm, and can even do good, if we're clear on what can and cannot be controlled.

- *We can't control other people.* Our children move away, our wives grow more and more independent, and even the people who work for us aren't ours. We can never know what they're thinking or planning; and if we base our lives on this impossible knowledge, we're in for stress of the most severe kind.

- *We can't control events.* Business decisions (and not even in our own business), government decisions (and not even of our own government) can have ripple effects that wash away a lifetime of expectations. A foreign steel mill lowers its prices, an American steel mill lays off some employees, there's less money to spend in the town—and the butcher's assistant is out of a job. If we base our sense of security on the premise that things are going to stay the way they are, we're setting ourselves up for shock after shock.

Insight alone is not enough. To change stress-producing perspectives and patterns, men must actually try out new actions and reactions, listen to new ideas and feedback, and then repeat the new approaches again and again. Living with stress requires, as I said in the Introduction, no less than a change in thinking, feelings, and behavior. And living without stress? To quote Hans Selye, father of stress research, "Complete freedom from stress is death." Let's choose life—a long, healthy, and happy life!

BIBLIOGRAPHY

ABERLE, D., and NAEGLE, K. "Middle Class Fathers' Occupational Role and Attitudes Toward Children." *American Journal of Orthopsychiatry* 22 (2) (1975): 366-378.

BANDURA, ALBERT; ROSS, D.; and ROSS, S. A. "Imitation of Film-Mediated Aggression Models." *Journal of Abnormal and Social Psychology* 63 (1961): 575-582.

———. "Transmission of Aggression Through Imitation of Aggressive Models." *Journal of Abnormal and Social Psychology* 63 (1961): 3-11.

BARRY, H.; BACON, M.; and CHILD, I. L. "A Cross-Cultural Survey of Some Sex Differences in Socialization." *Journal of Abnormal and Social Psychology* 92 (2): 119-133.

BECKER, J. B.; BREEDLOVE, S. M.; and CREWS, D. *Behavioral Endocrinology.* Cambridge, Mass.: The MIT Press, 1992.

BELL, DONALD. *Being a Man: The Paradox of Masculinity.* San Diego: Harcourt Brace Jovanovich, 1982.

BISHOP, J. E. "Bacterium Causes Most Peptic Ulcers." *The Wall Street Journal*, February 10, 1994.

BITTMAN, S., and ZALK, S. *Expectant Fathers.* New York: Hawthorne Books, 1978.

BLOTNICK, S. *The Corporate Steeplechase: Predictable Crises in a Business Career.* New York: Facts on File, 1984.

BOFFEY, P. M. "Satisfaction on the Job: Autonomy Ranks First." *The New York Times*, May 28, 1985.

BOWLBY, J. Quoted in "Leaving Marks Life Experiences, Measures Maturation, Stability," by D. Goleman. *The New York Times*, April 3, 1984.

BRAZELTON, T. B. "How Babies Handle Stress." *Redbook*, May 1983.

BURISH, T. G.; MAISTO, S. A.; and SHIRLEY, M. C. "Effect of Alcohol and Stress on Emotional and Physiological Arousal." *Motivation and Emotion* 6 (2): 149–159.

BURNETT, E. C., JR. "The Effects of Stress on Conflict Resolution Skills in Individuals from Violent Versus Nonviolent Families of Origin." Dissertation, University of Southern Mississippi, 1982.

CAPLAN, ROBERT, et al. "Job Demands and Worker Health." Washington, D.C.: National Institution for Occupational Safety and Health (Publication #75–160), April 1975.

CHARATRAN, FRED. Quoted in *Stress and Productivity*, S. Kieffer, ed. New York: Human Sciences Press, 1984.

CLEARY, E. J. Letter to the Editor. *The New York Times*, April 28, 1993.

CODDINGTON, R. D., and TROXELL, J. R. "The Effect of Emotional Factors on Football Injury Rates: A Pilot Study." *Journal of Human Stress* 6 (4) (1980): 3–5.

COMPAS, B. E. "Stress and Life Events During Childhood and Adolescence." *Clinical Psychology Review* 7 (1987): 175–302.

CONDRY, J. C., JR.; SIMAN, M. L.; and BONFRENBRENNER, U. "Characteristics of Peer-Adult-Oriented Children." Unpublished manuscript. Cited in *A Child's World*, by D. E. Papalia and S. W. Olds. New York: McGraw-Hill, 1979.

CORDES, C. "Kahneman: Loss Looms Large." American Psychological Association *Monitor*, December 1984.

COUSINS, N. *Anatomy of an Illness as Perceived by the Patient*. New York: W. W. Norton, 1979.

DIAGRAM GROUP. *Man's Body: A User's Manual*. New York: Bantam Books, 1976.

DIXON, S. *Working With People in Crisis*. St. Louis: C. V. Mosby, 1979.

ECKHOLM, E. "Value of Meditation Against Stress Now Questioned." *The New York Times*, July 24, 1984.

EDELSON, R. Quoted in "Severe Stress Seems to Be a Madison Avenue Pressure." *Adweek*, September 28, 1981.

EHRENREICH, B. *The Hearts of Men*. New York: Anchor/Doubleday, 1983.

ERIKSON, E. *Childhood and Society*. New York: W. W. Norton, 1963.

FISHER, K. "Berkeley Study Finds Stress Is Value-Laden." American Psychological Association *Monitor*, December 1984.

FISHER, STANLEY. *Discovering the Power of Self-Hypnosis*. New York: HarperCollins Publishers, 1991.

FRIEDMAN, M. Reported in "Count to 10 and Pet the Dog," by L. Mansnerus. *The New York Times*, April 25, 1993.

FRIEDMAN, M., and ROSENMAN, R. *Type A Behavior and Your Heart*. New York: Alfred A. Knopf, 1974.

FRIEDMAN, M., and ULMER, D. *Treating Type A Behavior and Your Heart*. New York: Alfred A. Knopf, 1984.

FRIEDMAN, R., ed. *Male Infancy-Childhood: Sex Differences in Behavior*. New York: Wiley & Sons, 1974.

GINOTT, H. *Between Parent and Child*. New York: Macmillan, 1965.

GLASSER, M. A. "Labor Looks at Work Stress." In *Stress and Productivity*, S. Kieffer, ed. New York: Human Sciences Press, 1984.

GLICK, I., et al. *The First Year of Bereavement*. New York: Wiley & Sons, 1974.

GOLEMAN, D. "Hope Seen for Curbing Youth Violence." *The New York Times*, August 11, 1993.

GOVE, W., and TUDOR, J. "Adult Sex Roles and Mental Illness." *American Journal of Sociology* 78 (4) (1973): 50-73.

GUNN, R. C. "Smoking Clinic Failures and Recent Life Stress." *Addictive Behavior* 8 (1) (1983): 83-87.

HARRAGAN, B. L. *Games Mother Never Taught Me*. New York: Warner Books, 1978.

HETHERINGTON, E. M. "Sex Typing, Dependency and Aggression." In *Perspectives in Child Psychology: Research Review*, T. D. Spenser and N. Kass, eds. New York: McGraw-Hill, 1970.

HIRSCHFELD, M. Quoted in "Relationships: Success and Guilt Feelings," by A. Brooks. *The New York Times*, July 21, 1984.

HOLMES, T. H., and RAHE, R. H. "The Social Readjustment Rating Scale." *Journal of Psychosomatic Research* 11 (1967): 213-221.

HOYT, M. Reported in "Treating Distress in Eight to Twenty Weeks," by N. Peterson. *USA Today*, December 7, 1984.

HUNT, M. "Research Through Deception." *The New York Times Magazine*, September 12, 1982.

HYER, K., and BUTLER, R. N. "Living Alone." *Merck Manual of Geriatrics*, 2nd ed. Rahway, N.J.: Merck Sharp & Dohme, 1994.

JAMES, S. A.; HARNETT, S. A.; and KALSBECK, W. D. "John Henryism and Blood Pressure Differences Among Black Men." *Journal of Behavioral Medicine* 6 (3) (1983): 259-278.

JEMMOTT, J. "Academic Stress, Power Motivation and Decrease in Secretion Rate of Salivatory Secretory Immunoglobulin A." *The Lancet*, June 15, 1978.

JUNG, C. Quoted in *Seasons of a Man's Life*, by D. J. Levinson. New York: Alfred A. Knopf, 1978.

KAGAN, J. *Personality Development*. New York: Harcourt Brace Jovanovich, 1971.

KAHNEMAN, D., and TVERSKY, A. Reported in "Kahneman: Loss Looms Large," by C. Cordes. American Psychological Association *Monitor*, December 1984.

KIEFFER, S. N., ed. *Stress and Productivity*. "Problems of Industrial Psychiatric Medicine" series. New York: Human Sciences Press, 1984.

KILEY, D. *The Peter Pan Syndrome: Men Who Never Grow Up*. New York: Dodd, Mead, 1983.

KIMURA, D. "Sex Differences in the Brain." *Scientific American*, 1992: 119–125.

KORN/FERRY INTERNATIONAL. *Decade of the Executive Woman*. New York: Korn/Ferry International, 1993.

KRENZ, E. W., and EDWARDS, S. W. "Effects of Hypnosis on State Anxiety and Stress in Male and Female Intercollegiate Athletes." *International Journal of Clinical and Experimental Hypnosis* 30 (2): 189–230.

KÜBLER-ROSS, E. *On Death and Dying*. New York: Macmillan, 1969.

LA MANNA, M. A., and RIEDMAN, A. *Marriages and Families*. Belmont, Calif.: Wadsworth, 1981.

LEVINSON, D. J. *Seasons of a Man's Life*. New York: Alfred A. Knopf, 1978.

LEWIS, M., et al. "Early Sex Differences in the Human: Studies of Socio-Economic Development." *Archives of Sexual Behavior* 4 (1975): 329–335.

LIEBERT, R. M. "Television and Social Learning." In *Television and Social Behavior* 11, J. P. Murray, E. A. Rubinstein, and G. A. Comstock, eds. Washington, D.C.: U.S. Government Printing Office, 1972.

LOVALLO, W. R., et al. "Work Pressure and the Type A Behavior Pattern Exam Stress in Male Medical Students." *Psychosomatic Medicine* 48 (1986): 125–133.

LYNN, D. *The Father: His Role in Child Development*. Monterey, Calif.: Brooks/Cole, 1974.

MATHENY, K. B., and CUPP, P. "Control, Desirability, and Anticipation as Moderating Variables Between Life Changes and Illness." *Journal of Human Stress* 9 (2) (1983): 14–23.

MATTHEWS, G. Quoted in "Therapist Finds Many Achievers Feel They're Fakes," by D. Goleman. *The New York Times*, September 1, 1984.

MATZ, M. Quoted in *Helping Clients with Special Concerns*, by S. Eisenberg and L. Patterson. Chicago: Rand McNally, 1979.

McCLELLAND, D., and PILON, D. *Journal of Personality and Social Psychology* 44 (3).

McCOY, K. *Coping with Teenage Depression*. New York: New American Library, 1982.

MEAD, M. *Male and Female: Study of the Sexes in a Changing World*. New York: Morrow, 1979.

MELAMED, S.; HARARI, G.; and GREEN, M. S. "Type A Behavior, Tension, and Ambulatory Cardiovascular Reactivity in Workers Exposed to Noise Stress." *Psychosomatic Medicine* 55 (1993): 185–192.

MEYER, J., and SOBIESZEK, B. "Effects of a Child's Sex on Adult Interpretations of Its Behavior." *Developmental Psychology* 6 (1972): 42–48.

MONEY, J., and EHRHARDT, A. *Man and Woman, Boy and Girl*. Baltimore: Johns Hopkins University Press, 1972.

MURDOCCO, R. Quoted in "On the Farm, Stress Grows Like a Weed," by D. Ketcham. *The New York Times*, January 31, 1993.

MUSSEN, P., and DISTLER, L. "Masculinity, Identification and Father–Son Relationships." *Journal of Abnormal and Social Psychology* 59 (1959).

NATIONAL INSTITUTE ON ALCOHOL ABUSE AND ALCOHOLISM. *Eighth Special Report to the U.S. Congress on Alcohol and Health from the Secretary of Health and Human Services*. Washington, D.C.: National Institutes of Health (NIH Pub. #94-3699), 1993.

New York Times, The. "Postal Study Aims to Spot Violence-Prone Workers." July 2, 1993.

NIEBERG, H. Quoted in "Combatting Stress for the Unemployed," by P. Singer. *The New York Times*, January 24, 1993.

PAPALIA, D. E., and OLDS, S. W. *A Child's World*. New York: McGraw-Hill, 1979.

PHILLIPS, D. P.; VAN VOORHEES, C. A.; and RUTH, T. E. "The Birthday: Lifeline or Deadline?" *Psychosomatic Medicine* 54 (1992): 532–542.

PUBLIC POLICY INSTITUTE (American Association of Retired Persons). *Changing Needs for Long-Term Care: A Chartbook*. Washington, D.C.: AARP, 1989.

ROGERS, C. *Client-Centered Therapy*. Boston: Houghton-Mifflin, 1951.

ROHSENOW, D. J. "Social Anxiety, Daily Moods, and Alcohol Use Over Time Among Heavy Social Drinkers." *Addictive Behavior* 7 (3) (1982): 311–315.

ROSENFIELD, S. "The Costs of Sharing: Wives' Employment and Husbands' Mental Health." *Journal of Health and Social Behavior* 33 (1992): 213–225.

RUBIN, S.; PROVENZANO, F.; and LURIA, Z. "The Eye of the Beholder: Parents' View on Sex of Newborns." *American Journal of Orthopsychiatry* 44 (4) (1974): 512–519.

RUBIN, Z. *Living and Loving*. New York: Holt, Rinehart & Winston, 1973.

RUOCCO, J. N. "Stress—How Useful a Concept." In *Stress and Productivity*, S. Kieffer, ed. New York: Human Sciences Press, 1984.

SADKER, M., and SADKER, D. *Failing at Fairness*. New York: Charles Scribner's Sons, 1994.

Sapolsky, R. M.; Krey, L. C.; and McEwen, B. S. "The Neuroendocrinology of Stress and Aging: The Glucocorticoid Cascade Hypothesis." *Endocrine Reviews* 7 (3) (1986): 284–301.

Schaie, K. W. Reported in "Mental Decline in Aging Need Not Be Inevitable," by D. Goleman. *The New York Times*, April 26, 1994.

Sedgwick, H. Quoted in "Relationships: Success and Guilt Feeling," by A. Brooks. *The New York Times*, July 21, 1984.

———. *The Stress of Life*, rev. ed. New York: McGraw-Hill, 1984.

Selye, H. *Stress Without Distress.* New York: Signet, 1974.

"Sex After Sixty: Plateaus, Not Valleys." *Science News,* October 17, 1981.

Sherman, J.; Harnett, S.; and Kalsbeek, w. "John Henryism and Blood Pressure Differences Among Black Men." *Journal of Behavioral Medicine* 6 (3) (September 1983).

Silverstein, o. Quoted in "Apron Strings Should Be Cut with Care," by N. Peterson. *USA Today,* December 4, 1984

Siman, M. "Application for a New Model of Peer Group Influence to Naturally Existing Adolescent Friendship Groups." *Child Development* 48 (1977): 270–274.

Steptoe, A.; Fieldman, G.; Evans, O.; and Perry, L. "Control Over Work Pace, Job Strain and Cardiovascular Responses in Middle-Aged Men." *Journal of Hypertension*, 11 (1993): 751–759.

Suarez, E. C., and Williams, R. B., Jr., "The Relationships Between Dimensions of Hostility and Cardiovascular Reactivity as a Function of Task Characteristics." *Psychosomatic Medicine* 51 (1989): 404–418.

Turner, J. R.; Sherwood, A.; and Light, K. C. *Individual Differences in Cardiovascular Response to Stress.* New York: Plenum Press, 1992.

"Type A: A Change of Heart and Mind." *Science News,* August 18, 1984.

U.S. Department of Commerce, Bureau of the Census. *Sixty-Five Plus in America. Current Population Reports, P23-178 RV.* Washington, D.C.: U.S. Government Printing Office, 1993.

U.S. Senate Special Committee on Aging, et al. *Aging America, Trends and Projections.* DHHS Pub. #(FCOA) 91–28001. Washington, D.C.: U.S. Government Printing Office, 1991.

Vaillant, G. E. *Adaptation to Life.* Boston: Little, Brown, 1979.

Van Egeren, L. F., and Sparrow, A. W. "Ambulatory Monitoring to Assess Real-Life Cardiovascular Reactivity in Type A and Type B Subjects." *Psychosomatic Medicine* 52 (1990): 297–306.

Vaux, A., and Ruggiero, M. "Stressful Life Change and Delinquent Behavior." *American Journal of Contemporary Psychology* 11 (2) (1983): 169–181.

Visotsky, H. M. "Socio-Cultural Aspects of Stress." In *Stress and Productivity*, S. Kieffer, ed. New York: Human Sciences Press, 1984.

WALTERS, J. "Coming to Terms After Years Apart." *USA Today*, June 29, 1985.

WARR, P., and PAYNE, R. "Affective Outcomes of Paid Employment in a Random Sample of British Workers." *Journal of Occupational Behavior (U.S.)* 4 (2) (1983): 91–104.

WARSHAW, L. J. "Managing Stress." In *Stress and Productivity*, S. Kieffer, ed. New York: Human Sciences Press, 1984.

WEIDNER, G.; HUTT, J.; CONNOR, S. L.; and MENDELL, N. R. "Family Stress and Coronary Risk in Children." *Psychosomatic Medicine* 54 (1992): 471–479.

WEINBERGER, D. A.; SCHWARTZ, G. E.; and DAVIDSON, R. J. "Low-Anxious, High-Anxious, and Repressive Coping Styles: Psychometric Patterns and Behavioral and Physiological Responses to Stress." *Journal of Abnormal Psychology* 88 (4) (1979): 369–380.

WEITZMAN, L.; EIFLER, D.; HOKADA, E.; and ROSS, C. "Sex-Role Socialization in Picture Books for Preschool Children." Quoted in *A Child's World*, by D. E. Papalia and S. W. Olds. New York: McGraw-Hill, 1979.

WILLIAMS, J. A., et al. "Sex Role Socialization in Picture Books: An Update." *Social Science Quarterly* 68 (1) (1987): 148–56.

WILLIAMS, R. B., et al. "Type A Behavior and Angiographically Documented Coronary Atherosclerosis in a Sample of 2,289 Patients." *Psychosomatic Medicine* 50 (1988): 139–152.

WINES, M. "Reno Chastises TV Networks on Violence in Programming." *The New York Times*, October 21, 1993.

WITKIN, M. H., and LEHRENBAUM, B. *Forty-five and Single Again*. New York: Dembner Books, 1985.

WOLKERS, M. "Eight Ways to Get Rid of a Headache." *Gannett Westchester Newspapers*, February 13, 1984.

INDEX

ABOUT THE AUTHOR

Georgia Witkin, Ph.D., is an assistant clinical professor of psychiatry and director of the stress program at the Mount Sinai School of Medicine in New York City. She served on the editorial boards of the *Journal of Preventive Psychology* and *Health* and authored several books including *The Female Stress Syndrome, Beyond Quick Fixes,* and *Passions.* In addition to her private psychotherapy practice, Dr. Witkin is a weekly contributor to *Today in New York,* and has her own nightly segment on WNBC-TV's *Live at Five.* Dr. Witkin is also a nationally known lecturer, has written and hosted her own television program *Just Between the Sexes* on CNBC, and has been the guest expert on more than 100 shows including *20/20, The Today Show, Live with Regis and Kathy Lee, The Don Imus Show,* and CNN. Her articles and comments have appeared in *Time Magazine, Parade, Newsweek, The New York Times, Men's Health, Newsweek,* and many other periodicals. Dr. Witkin lives in New York City.

STRESS MANAGEMENT BOOKS FROM NEWMARKET PRESS

The Female Stress Syndrome—Second Edition
How to Become Stress-Wise in the '90s
Georgia Witkin, Ph.D.

Dr. Witkin reveals how and why women experience stress differently than men. Included are checklists, quizzes, and a female stress questionnaire to help women identify sources of stress in their personal and public lives. Dr. Witkin identifies the symptoms of stress overload and provides practical, short- and long-term coping strategies.

The Male Stress Syndrome—Second Edition
How to Become Stress-Wise in the '90s
Georgia Witkin, Ph.D.

Dr. Witkin explains why men develop the stress symptoms they do; how stress affects their bodies, careers, families, personal goals and expectations; and the differences between men and women coping with stress. She outlines the early warning signs of potentially harmful stress; provides checklists and profiles so that men can rate their own stress levels; and offers simple effective stress management strategies.

Stressmap: Personal Diary Edition—Expanded Edition
The Ultimate Stress Management, Self-Assessment and Coping Guide
Developed by Essi Systems. Foreword by Robert K. Cooper, Ph.D.

This stress measurement tool used by more than 1,500 companies, hospitals, and colleges gives you a revealing portrait of your stress health. The self-scoring questionnaire poses 300 questions about your environment, your inner world, your coping responses, and your own signals of stress overload. The "Action Planning Guide" gives more than 100 effective strategies for handling pressure on the job and at home.